THE RUNNER'S
YOGA BOOK

THE RUNNER'S
YOGA BOOK

A BALANCED APPROACH
TO FITNESS

Jean Couch

RODMELL
PRESS

Berkeley, California
1990

Library of Congress Catalog Card Number: 90–70758

ISBN 0-9627138-1-3

Linda Cogozzo Donald Moyer
Editors

Katherine L. Kaiser
Copy Editor

Andrea DuFlon
DuFlon Design Associates
Designer

Chris Orr
Production Artist

Fred Stimson
Cover Photographer

David Madison
Photographer

Ellen Sasaki
Illustrator

McNaughton & Gunn, Inc.
Saline, Michigan
Lithographer

Text set in Adobe Stone Serif and ITC Avant Garde
03 02 01 00   10 11 12 13

To Janie

CONTENTS

Acknowledgments

I wish to acknowledge

First, the Grace that gave me the opportunity to write this book. I have enjoyed the experience enormously!

Second, the ultimate source of this information, B.K.S. Iyengar of Pune, India. I have unlimited respect for his genius and overflowing gratitude for his willingness to share it.

In addition, Nell Weaver of Little Rock, Arkansas, for her bountiful contributions, editorial and otherwise. Behind this author is an excellent contributor. And Nell wishes to thank her teacher, Janet Downs.

Also, my teachers: Ramanand Patel and the other teachers at the Iyengar Yoga Institute (formerly the Institute for Yoga Teacher Education) in San Francisco: Felicity Hall, Mary Dunn, Larry Hatlett, Melinda Perlee, Bonita Bradley, Toni Montez, Judith Lasater, and Bridget Gleason.

And, all my students. Each person brings his or her own mystery. Every person is an education.

Further, Dr. Gary Harper of Little Rock, Arkansas, for reading the physiology section. Emily Stuart of Los Altos, California, for reviewing Part One, "The Basics" section.

Finally, my family. Whitney, age three, who helped so much with her secretarial skills: sharpening pencils, walking on chapters, stapling everything in sight. Matthew, age six, who left a jar of worms on my desk and held steadfast in his belief that indeed this would one day be over so we could go to the park again. Michael, husband, lover, friend, who pulled us all through with his even disposition, good humor, and generosity. My Mom and Dad, Iva and Bill McWilliams, who spent all those years helping me prepare for such a satisfying project as this.

Acknowledgments for the Revised Edition

I wish to acknowledge

Angela Farmer, who gave me back my breath and the ability to see spring.

Angie Thusius, for coming into my life at just the right moment.

John Smolowe, for eternal patience, optimism, and lovingkindness.

Linda Cogozzo and Donald Moyer, for encouragement and enormous support.

And again Michael, Matthew, and Whitney, always and forever the ultimate teachers and lovers.

Preface

Here I am writing the first words last. It's wonderful to write a book because you can "let it rip" and say so many things you've always wanted to say. I wish I could include a dehydrated capsule with this: You add the water and out would come a miniature teacher. One to cajole you, to direct you, to encourage you, to teach you yoga. One who would work you when you babied yourself. One to hold you back when you pushed too hard. One who had so much love and respect for you and for yoga that by his or her talents he or she helped you discover yourself.

But because I can't include this ultimate gimmick, I ask you to draw upon your imagination as you use this book. The pictures are static, the directions are precise, the intent is serious. But don't let the medium kill the humanity of it all. There will be times when you will want to laugh, cry, curse, quit. Do all of these things but then return. Return to the poses in this book, and bit by bit you will indeed become flexible.

Flexibility is the ability to change: the ability to see and adjust, see and adjust, see and adjust. Although Hatha Yoga teaches flexibility through the concreteness of the body, the flexibility you gain will be much more than physical.

I wish I could shower you with my enthusiasm, to give you the spark of interest that would lead you to the discoveries possible through the practice of this scientific art form of the body, mind, spirit: yoga!

Jean Couch
Los Altos Hills, California
March 1979

Preface to the Revised Edition

Here I am, ten years later returning to *The Runner's Yoga Book* (formerly *Runner's World Yoga Book*). I am grateful so many found this book useful the first time and I wanted to write a revised edition to provide an update of my understanding of the techniques of Iyengar yoga. I honor and appreciate the brilliant teachings of B.K.S. Iyengar.

Jean Couch
Los Altos Hills, California
September 1989

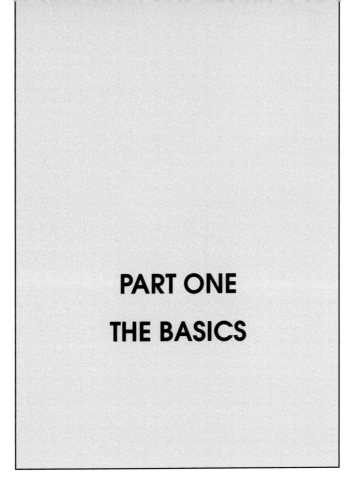

PART ONE

THE BASICS

1
EASTERN YOGA FOR THE WESTERN ATHLETE

The specialized ways of the Western world have so thoroughly dissected the human being that it is common to accept false divisions of the human being into body, mind, and spirit. The emphasis on intellectual pursuits accompanied by neglect of both body and spirit are manifestations of the assumption that happiness can be accomplished through the head alone. But signs of dissatisfaction with this situation are everywhere visible. Self-help and consciousness-raising groups that nurture the spirit are flourishing. The importance of physical fitness has come to be more and more appreciated. These new waves of enthusiasm reflect an attempt to more thoroughly integrate the body with the mind and the spirit. The East has dealt with this issue for centuries. Those who wish to realize their own wholeness can turn to yoga.

The word *yoga* means "union" or "joining." There are numerous systems of yoga, each providing different ways to unify the various aspects of the human being. The yoga system this book deals with is Hatha Yoga. In the simplest terms Hatha Yoga means "yoga for health"; it is the physical aspect of yoga. The Sanskrit word *hatha* implies balance: *ha* means "sun" and *tha* means "moon." This system of yoga aims to balance—to join—different energy flows within the human body.

3

Hatha Yoga is the system most familiar to the Westerner. It works through the concreteness of the body. Hatha Yoga uses physical poses (asanas) to explore the inner structures of the body, the mind, and the spirit. It is a path, a guide, a step-by-step method that can lead you to greater self-knowledge. Each pose is a means to feel inwardly, to discover where you are strong, tight, weak, or dull. Thus, Hatha Yoga provides a framework for the experiences of physical, mental, and spiritual wholeness.

Within the system of Hatha Yoga there are numerous approaches. The poses in this book are based, for the most part, on the teaching of B.K.S. Iyengar, author of the classic text, *Light on Yoga* (New York: Schocken, 1979), *Light on Pranayama* (New York: Crossroad, 1981), and *The Tree of Yoga* (Boston: Shambhala, 1989). Now in his seventies, Iyengar teaches primarily at his institute, The Ramamani Iyengar Memorial Yoga Institute, in Pune, India. He has spent more than fifty years practicing and developing the art of yoga. His approach emphasizes precise and careful body alignment, muscular balance, and maximum spinal extension.

The Iyengar method of yoga is based on a central principle of balance. Physiologically balance means several things:

- Each individual muscle is capable of contracting, lengthening, and relaxing.
- Corresponding muscle groups (for example, hamstrings and quadriceps) are equally strengthened and stretched.
- The joints, when surrounded by balanced muscle tissues, are free to move in their full range of motion.
- Alignment of the body makes it possible to accommodate a full breath.
- Energy flows equally to all parts of the body.

Therefore, the Iyengar approach to yoga is a science of postural work highly useful to the Western athlete.

When the body is balanced, flesh feels like flesh; it is neither too hard (and susceptible to injury) nor too soft (and incapable of supporting the skeleton properly). When the body is balanced, the musculoskeletal system facilitates movement, rather than hinders it. The body is designed for nothing if not for movement, and balanced movement is self-perpetuating: the more freely you move, the more you can move.

In my opinion Iyengar's approach to Hatha Yoga promotes this balance better than any other school of Hatha Yoga or any fitness program presently available. His system teaches how to move the spine to preserve and strengthen its natural integrity. And what's most helpful is that the work is individual: no matter what your particular imbalances or problems are, Iyengar yoga will teach you how to move in the way most appropriate for you.

And the marvel of it all is that it works through the concreteness of the body. You don't have to change your religious beliefs to experience the benefits of Hatha Yoga. The one thing you must do is practice the poses. The means to physical, mental, and spiritual wholeness are your own body in the poses and your own willingness to observe closely how you feel. Athletes are already working with their bodies; what many need to do is learn a new way to look and to feel in order to bring about a more satisfying harmony that comes not only from physical equilibrium but from mental and spiritual balance as well.

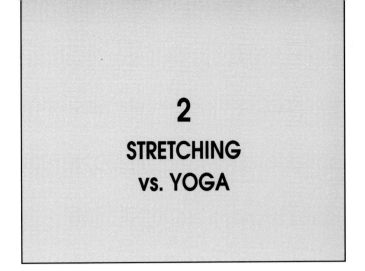

2
STRETCHING
vs. YOGA

Dynamic stretching differs from yoga stretching, or static stretching, in process and purpose. Dynamic stretching is jerky and forced; yoga stretching is slow and controlled. Dynamic stretching aims for a certain degree of flexibility; yoga stretching aims for physical, mental, and spiritual balance.

Dynamic stretching means that a person bounces or jerks into a certain position. The completed stretch is seldom held for more than a few seconds. The intention is to achieve a predetermined degree of flexibility. This method of stretching is an attempt by the mind to force the body into an idealized form. The brain tries to dictate to the body. There is little dialogue between the body and the mind; only the most intense feelings are heeded. Those engaged in this activity may be spurred on by what they see someone else do or by what someone else expects, often comparing themselves with others or with goals others have set for them. Stretching in such cases is competitive.

In yoga stretching, a person uses a slow, steady motion to enter a pose, holding at the limit of his or her stretch for ten seconds to ten minutes, or longer. The slowness of yoga gives the practitioner greater control over the positioning, safety, and efficiency of each pose. Yoga is introspective, allowing the practitioner to look within and to feel how he or she responds physically and emotionally to the poses. The precision necessary for each pose guides the practitioner to physical balance. For example, in any given standing pose, the outer muscles of the leg work equally to those of the inner leg; the inside of the foot bears as much weight as the outside of the foot. The lower body may be supporting the torso, but the upper body is not passive. It is alive and complements the alignment of the lower body. When doing yoga, attention is given to the front of the body as well as to the back; to the sides, the limbs, the joints, the muscles; to the flow of energy; to the breath.

But yoga can produce this physical balance only if the mind and body cooperate. This entails two elements: locating imbalances and then adjusting them. While doing each pose the mind must be receptive to the messages the body is sending. Once the messages are understood, an adjustment can be made.

This intimate interplay between the body and the mind is the essence of yoga, and the essential difference between yoga stretching and dynamic stretching. Balance requires precise attention. Doing yoga is similar to walking a tightrope: you are never stationary, but always adjusting to the movement of the rope. You cannot come to inner balance and be fully present in a pose if your mind wanders to the grocery list, the house assessment, social entanglements, or the person next to you. Not that the mind doesn't do that; for it to do so is the very nature of mind. But when it does wander off, you can restore balance in the pose by gently drawing the mind back "into" the body.

So the static stretching of yoga is very different from dynamic stretching. The degree of flexibility achieved does not determine success in yoga. Success is measured by your inward attention to the body and mind in the pose. No matter how flexible you are, yoga is accessible to you; it's simply a matter of being willing to feel and respond to yourself.

3
RATIONALE
AND RESULTS

As an athlete you can benefit from yoga in three major ways. Because yoga is an effective way to both stretch and strengthen the body, it promotes physical balance, increases mental alertness, and helps to prevent injuries and discomforts. Furthermore, learning to use the body in this more efficient way is likely to improve your athletic performance.

When you feel refreshed and attentive after exercise, it is because activity has stimulated the action of the muscles in pumping fluids through the body. More efficient pumping by the muscles depends on their level of elasticity. Such elasticity will increase through the practice of yoga. In the same way increased muscular flexibility and strength will prevent many common injuries and annoyances (for example, muscle pulls and stiffness) that strenuous exercise can cause.

To understand how yogic stretching can accomplish these results, it is important to know how your body functions and moves. The next few pages present this basic information and discuss the ways in which yoga can influence this functioning for better health and improved athletic performance.

The Physiological Case for Yoga Stretching
The power for athletic movement is produced by the contraction, or shortening, of muscles. Stretching

can counteract the negative effects (detailed in this chapter) of the repeated contractions that occur during running and other sports. For example, when you bend your forearm, it is the contraction of the biceps (upper arm muscles) that draws up the arm. To reverse the action of the arm in straightening the elbow, the contraction of the opposing muscles, the triceps, must occur. During this latter contraction, the biceps lengthen, but only to accommodate the contraction of the triceps. The muscles act as a lever, and the joints as a fulcrum, when muscles contract. Movement is the result of muscles shortening; muscles pull bones together rather than pushing bones apart.

All athletic exertion, then, can be viewed as the repetitive and coordinated contraction of muscles and muscle groups. Such continual contractions determine the resting length of the muscle spindle, the message center of the muscle. When the spindle learns that the muscle is continually being asked to shorten, it adjusts to the demands placed upon it and becomes increasingly resistant to stretching or lengthening. Muscles that are persistently worked without stretching can thus become hard and short.

These bulging muscles conform to our culture's traditional view of health and strength, but they are not pliable or adaptable. Stiff muscles deprive the body of optimum health by

- Inhibiting the movement of joints
- Prohibiting the full contraction of opposing muscles
- Misaligning the body
- Decreasing body efficiency
- Increasing the possibility of injury
- Deterring the maximum pumping action within each muscle

• Inhibiting the movement of joints. This potential difficulty is exemplified by what can happen to the hip joint. You probably spend a lot of time sitting—at the office, in your car, in front of the television—which causes the muscles that draw the thighs up to the torso (hip flexors) to shorten and no longer accommodate full movement in the hip socket. (This joint is a ball in a socket, and is capable of a wide range of motion.) If the muscles at the front of the hip joint are shortened, the leg is not able to move backward as far as it once could. The thighbone is no longer being moved fully in the socket. This then retards the flow of synovial fluid, which lubricates the joints, and the chances of calcium buildup increase. Tightened hip flexors also contribute to swayback, in which the front of the pelvis is pulled down.

•**Prohibiting the full contraction of opposing muscles.** All muscles work in pairs. For example, as the hip flexors draw the thigh up to the torso, the hamstring and buttock muscles lengthen. Conversely, when the leg is moved backward, the hip flexors lengthen as the hamstrings and buttocks shorten. But if the hip flexors are too tight and cannot lengthen fully, their opposing muscles cannot contract completely. Muscles or portions of muscles that are not worked lose strength and tone and are less able to move the skeleton properly.

•**Misaligning the body.** All muscles act as levers, and shortened muscles can pull the body out of alignment. In general, muscles are designed to move the body and bones are designed to support the body. When bones are stacked up correctly—like building blocks—they are in balance with gravity, or aligned. The spine is in alignment when it has four long, gentle curves; the neck and lower back have concave curves, the tailbone area and rib cage area have convex curves. However, tight muscles can pull bones out of alignment. For example, tight abdominal muscles pull the sternum down, causing a collapse in the chest and a humping in the rib cage area of the spine (kyphosis). The neck also shortens. Now, instead of the body balancing on bones with a minimum of effort, numerous muscles and ligaments must contract to work against the pull of gravity pull. This necessitates a greater output of energy just to remain upright, and creates tension in the body, which inhibits the vital functions of digestion, circulation, and breathing.

•**Decreasing body efficiency.** Stiffness of muscles and joints is often caused by muscles that are permanently shortened through strengthening without stretching (or through gross inactivity). This stiffness is a drain on the body's energy, for muscles use energy to remain semicontracted. Also, when a muscle is continually contracted, it cannot lengthen to accommodate the contraction of its opposing muscle. This means that the brain, which receives the major portion of its sensory information from the muscles, is receiving confusing messages. When the brain receives a message to contract a muscle, the message is muddled if the opposing muscle cannot lengthen fully.

•Increasing the possibility of injury. When a joint is surrounded by tight, shortened muscles, the body is structurally susceptible to harm. If a muscle does not move freely, the joint may move without it, causing a dislocation or a torn ligament, tendon, or muscle. Injury can also occur simply from chronic shortening. For example, if the hamstrings are continually shortened, as they are in running, they can compress the hip joint or knee joint. Such compression can lead to torn cartilage, pain in the hip, sciatica, or rotation at the knee.

•Deterring the maximum pumping action within each muscle. Muscle action may be compared to a sponge. When the sponge is squeezed, which is the equivalent of a muscle contracting, fluids flow. But for the sponge to absorb fluids efficiently again, it must be released and soft. So it is with muscles. If they are to pump efficiently, they must be able to contract to move fluids onward, and then soften again to absorb the fluids they require.

It is important that anyone who has embarked on a fitness plan be aware of the preceding facts, and understand that there is a simple preventative solution: yoga.

Dynamic stretching, which is not used in yoga, actually shortens a muscle. The simple kneejerk reflex is a good example of this. This reflex protects the muscles and surrounding joints from overstretching when they have been stretched too far or too fast beyond their resting length.

Static stretching, the stretching of yoga, involves positioning the body so that a muscle or muscle group is stretched, and then holding in this position. The static stretch increases the resting length of a muscle and thereby enhances resiliency. To bring about relaxation after sustained shortening activities, a muscle should be held in a stretch position so that the cortex of the brain can first receive information about the stretch and then send out new instructions to the muscle spindle to lengthen.

Static stretching enhances your capacity to be sensitive to how you feel. Excessive muscular tightness means that the brain is always receiving messages from the stretch reflex system. Such tightness makes the muscles very sensitive to stretching. When a muscle is chronically tight simple movements such as walking are perceived as stretches. This causes the reflex system to contract that muscle much more often than a resilient muscle. This continual stimulation of the brain makes it less sensitive to subtler messages from the body. When the resting length of muscles is increased, the stretch reflex is not elicited as often, thus permitting the brain to receive and respond to other stimuli.

Static stretching also increases body strength. When you are stretching one muscle, its opposite muscle must be contracting. This muscle that is contracting probably has been weakened and has lost tone because it has been accommodating its antagonist muscle which is overly tight. Such weakening impairs the ability of the muscle to function properly.

True fitness, then, is more than just strength. Pure strength is an important component of fitness; it provides stability and power. But flexibility is also crucial for adaptability. Genuine fitness means achieving a balance between strength and flexibility.

For most people, fitness is something over which they have control. By their chosen activities they can improve their health by doing more of what makes them feel better and less of what isn't beneficial. Although stretching is difficult at the outset, perseverance will be rewarded. All athletes, who are committed to a health-giving regimen, can benefit from the greater bodily strength and flexibility—in short, more complete and well-rounded fitness and health—that regular yoga practice can bring.

4
GETTING STARTED

You've read about why to do yoga. Let's now discuss how to get started with your yoga practice. You may or may not have a teacher. If not, how do you select one? If you're not interested in a teacher or don't have access to one, how do you proceed on your own? How can this book help you?

With or Without a Teacher

Yoga traditionally has been passed on from teacher to student. It is the best way to learn yoga. Teachers can often see what you can't. It is very difficult to see habitual imbalances embedded in your own body and mind. Because these aberrations feel normal, you aren't even aware of your unawareness. By offering the perspective of an interested and educated outsider, the teacher can be a catalyst for increased awareness of your body.

If you are interested in studying yoga with a teacher, I suggest you try to find one who teaches the Iyengar method of yoga (see Chapter 25, "Resources"). Find out if the person practices yoga regularly; the poses demonstrated during class don't count. He or she should be trained in anatomy and kinesiology. And, of course, each teacher has his or her own style. Find one who is appropriate to your likes, dislikes, and needs.

If you have a teacher, this book can reinforce the

information presented in class and assist you in your practice at home. If you choose to work on your own—and it is possible to do so—the following information can serve to guide you.

Yoga on Your Own

•**When to do yoga.** Regularity is the key to your yoga practice. Find some time in your day that you will have available regularly—maybe before or after your athletic workout, perhaps first thing in the morning. You really should practice six days out of seven, but if that seems excessive, begin with every other day or four days a week. It's best not to eat for two hours before practice.

•**Duration.** In the beginning do yoga for fifteen to twenty minutes at each practice session. As your interest grows you will find that you naturally extend the time. For total balance practice yoga equally as long as you do athletic or other strenuous activities.

•**Setting.** Choose a clean, flat area where you can practice undisturbed. Do not work in direct sunlight. You will need one or more firm blankets or a mat.

•**Clothing.** Look at your shoes. The heels and soles reflect, and therefore reinforce, all the imbalances in your body. You might slip if you wore socks. It is essential, therefore, that you work with bare feet. Wear loose, comfortable clothing; your workout clothes are perfect.

•**Beginning a pose.** First, meticulously follow the placement directions given for each pose. This information is the foundation for the pose, and the basis for the balancing effects of yoga. If you walk with your feet turned out and stretch with your feet turned out, you reinforce a misalignment. So pay close attention to the initial instructions. If the foundation is wrong, the benefits of the pose are lost.

•**Move into the pose slowly.** When movement is slow it is more difficult to harm yourself, because your body gradually moves to its limit and there is no momentum to push it into injury. When movement is slow you can more easily feel which muscles are working and which part of your body needs attention.

•**Do not bounce.** To bounce into a stretch activates the dynamic stretch reflex, the mechanism built into the muscles to prevent overstretching. To lengthen a muscle by bouncing or jerking makes it shorten automatically to protect itself from overstretching. So, although a person stretching this way may say, "But I feel it stretch," in fact, what he or she is actually feeling is resistance to the stretch. Forcing the body in this way can lead to injury.

•**How far should you go into the pose?** Go as far into the pose as you can while comfortably maintaining the alignment described. It is only beneficial to do the pose with correct alignment. You should be on the "edge" of your stretch, that is, feeling sensation but not pain. If you are complacent changes will not occur; if you are overly ambitious you will get hurt. Listen to your body.

•**Holding the pose.** Once in the pose hold it as long as your breath is even. In the beginning that might be for ten to fifteen seconds, or even less. As your body gains flexibility and strength, slowly begin to increase your time in the pose. You may want to add one complete breath (inhalation and exhalation) or two seconds or five seconds at a time until you reach the maximum time given for each pose.

•**Attention.** While in the pose turn all your attention inward and consider: How do I feel? How does my body respond to the structure of the pose? Where am I strong? Where do I feel fatigue? Where is my tightest spot? Does the pose elicit any emotion? What am I learning about myself? The possibilities are unending. Be receptive.

•**Breathe!** Never hold the breath; it tightens the body. Always breathe through the nose with the mouth closed. Use the breath to help you stretch by moving on slow, steady, quiet exhalations. (Exceptions to this use of exhalations are noted in the descriptions of the individual poses.)

•**Relaxation**. In all phases of your practice, eliminate extra effort. Activate those muscles necessary to hold the pose, but notice and release any tension in the eyes, face, neck, jaw, throat, shoulders, or stomach. These are the areas where muscles are most frequently contracted. Then watch for any other areas you may be unnecessarily contracting. Just knowing where you are holding will assist you to release.

•**Handling discomfort.** While holding a pose notice where in your body you feel the most unpleasant sensation. This is where the bind is. Many people deal with this type of discomfort by tightening the surrounding muscles in an attempt to protect the area. Tightening muscles around the area of discomfort simply locks it into your body. Instead try the following: While in the pose get to know this place in your body. Visualize what it might look like: How big is it? What shape is it? What color is it? Does it moan, fidget, jump, burn, or scream? Allow the bound area to change. Getting to know the bound area is a beginning to unlocking and releasing it. Observation is the initial stage of all change.

•**What about pain?** If you feel pain, come out the pose mindfully. Reread the instructions. Adjust the pose to lessen the stretch (perhaps you will need to return to one of the earlier stages suggested with each pose). Remember, overstretching is just as ineffective as understretching—neither has a place in a balanced yoga practice. Finally, seek the advice of a competent teacher if you are unable to eliminate a persistent pain.

•**Adjusting a pose.** When you feel the need to change a pose, make any changes from the ground up. In standing poses begin changes with the feet; in sitting poses begin with the sitting bones and placement of the pelvis; in inverted poses begin with the head, shoulders, and elbows. Then observe your body. Never assume anything. Even though you think you have placed your feet correctly, look at them and be sure. Make any necessary changes, and then do the pose again.

•**Competition is out.** Do not compete with yoga illustrations or photographs, your companion, your teacher, or yourself. Assess and accept your own stretching capacity. This capacity will change from day to day and from moment to moment. To be caught up in competition or athletic goals necessitates surrender of your inner awareness. When competition occurs in yoga, the joy of self-discovery remains elusive or simply disappears. And forcing a stretch can abuse or injure muscles, tendons, and ligaments. Work with your body and not with your ego.

•**Ending the pose.** Take care as you come out of a pose. As you move out of the pose, focus on your alignment and breathe as slowly and evenly as you did when assuming the position. Unless specific directions are given, come out of the pose in the same way you moved into it. In so doing, you contract the same muscles that were stretched. Sometimes you may fall or collapse out of a pose for one reason or another, but try not to do this. Abrupt posture changes will negate the strengthening that comes from proper movement and may also cause injury.

•**Working with imbalances.** You will probably notice that one side of your body responds differently than the other. You may feel stiffer, weaker, or duller on one side. Sometimes it may be helpful to do a pose twice on your dull side because this side needs more care and attention than your more responsive side. Also, bring balance to your body and practice by reviewing the poses in the book frequently. Do you avoid some poses? These may be the ones you need the most.

•**Working with an injury.** If you sustain an injury, continue doing poses that do not affect the injured area. When you have an injury, consult with your physician before stretching the injured area. Take this book to the doctor and show him or her what you intend to do. In general, when you have injury to muscles, ligaments, or tendons, you should not stretch the area for three weeks. This gives it time to heal. Begin stretching the injured area by doing the easiest pose for that area. If the pose causes pain, discontinue it for another week. If it does not cause pain, practice this one pose for two weeks. (It takes two to three weeks for a pose to affect the body.) If the area continues to improve after this time, add another pose. Do these two poses for two weeks and then add a third, and so on. (If you add more than one pose at a time, you will not know which pose is doing what.) Proper movement can be therapeutic if you work intelligently. Working this way may seem slow. Acknowledge your impatience but know that perseverance will pay off.

Practical Suggestions for Beginning Yoga

1. If you have a special condition (for example, abnormal blood pressure, a history of back pain or injury, pregnancy, and so on), please seek the advice of your physician and a qualified yoga teacher before proceeding.
2. Practice in a clean, well-lighted space. Set aside a few minutes each day when you can practice undisturbed. Fifteen to twenty minutes a day is usually adequate in the beginning. When doing these poses outside, be sure you are on level ground, away from direct sunlight, and far from the "madding crowd." This gives you a chance to respond more carefully to how you feel.
3. Wait at least two hours after eating before beginning your practice. Evacuate your bladder and bowels before stretching.

4. Wear comfortable clothing that will allow your body to move. Always practice barefoot.

5. Breathe quietly through the nose. Most of the major movements are done on an exhalation.

6. Soften the body and allow the brain to be alert and watchful. Keep your eyes open so you practice being in the outer world while attending to inner feelings. The occasional use of a full-length mirror can be very helpful to check your alignment and make adjustments.

7. Careful attention to your alignment is essential. Learn the placement instructions for each pose.

8. Do not become dependent on the aids. Work one day with them, the next day without them.

9. You will find you have a less challenging side and a more challenging side. Occasionally do the more challenging side twice.

10. The poses you resist the most are likely the ones you need the most.

11. Be persistent and energetic and, at the same time, be gentle and nonviolent toward yourself.

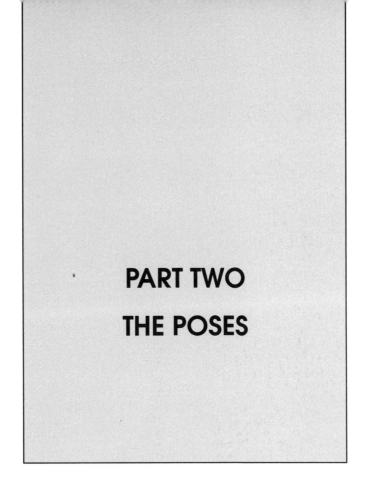

PART TWO

THE POSES

5
DIGGING IN

Part One of this book discusses information about yoga. Part Two details information about the poses themselves. The poses are demonstrated by three models, who vary in flexibility, strength, and yoga experience. They show how the poses can be adapted to meet different needs while working in the same general framework.

Don Nystrom runs forty miles a week and has limited (ten one-and-a-half-hour lessons) experience with yoga. His poses show how you might look in the beginning. Tim Durbin played football in college, runs about twenty-five miles a week, and has done yoga for a couple of years. Barbara Delisle Avery is a yoga practitioner and teacher and a runner. Scattered throughout this revised edition are recent photos of Tim and Barbara. Both of them continue to practice yoga and run. Barbara also runs after a two-year-old and works part-time; Tim chases golf balls, teaches school, and models.

The introduction to each chapter has important information on how to approach these particular poses. Some anatomical information is included to enhance your understanding of why it is best to move in a certain way. When a direction makes sense it is easier to do what's being asked, and to remember correct movement and positioning. In the introduction there are also general directions for all of these poses to avoid undue repetitions. These may be the most important directions, either for safety or for the effectiveness of the stretch. Please read them.

Be sure to begin with the poses in Chapter 6, "More Than Just Beginning: Preliminaries." The exercises may seem overly simple, but are basic to the instructions given for all subsequent poses.

For organizational purposes the poses are loosely categorized according to parts of the body. In a sense, though, this is a false division, because the body is a whole: while stretching the feet, the head is affected. Any forward bending pose stretches the entire back side, any backbending pose stretches the entire front side. So you may find that the best pose for you to stretch your knee may be in the chapter on hips and thighs. Bodies vary so much that you simply must do a wide variety of poses to see what affects you the most. You will then have become your own best teacher.

Within each category the poses are given in the approximate order of difficulty. This order of difficulty will not always be true for you, because the degree of difficulty depends on your body. No matter how flexible you think you are, do each pose in succession until you find one that really stretches you (but not to the point of pain). Maybe one of the easier poses is exactly the one that will affect a certain tight spot. Practice this one.

Experience will quickly show you where you should be working. You may find discrepancies. For example, you may be able to do the fifth hamstring stretch but only the first groin stretch. Follow your body's response.

For each pose I have divided the practice instructions as follows:

1. Placement
2. Pose
3. Variations
4. Aids

(Sometimes Preparation, rather than Pose, is the second entry, Pose is the third entry, and so on.)

The Placement section is very important. It provides the foundation and can make the difference between a stretch and a pose, and between reinforcing misalignments and correcting them. Follow these directions carefully.

Usually the complete pose follows the placement instructions. There may be times, however, when it is more appropriate for you to work with a variation or aid. I have shown the complete pose so you can see the framework in which you are working. With the exception of Shoulderstand (see Chapter 16) and Plough Pose (see Chapter 16), I frequently teach a pose by having people do the complete pose first. This gives them information about their tightnesses and weaknesses. Also, this way they appreciate the aid or variation more. So you too may begin with the completed pose. If you can maintain the alignment of the pose, then this is where you can work. However, do not dismiss the aids or variations. Often they can be guides to deeper understanding of the poses. If you can't maintain the alignment of the complete pose, then practice from the variations and aids sections.

Variations show you how to do the pose with some modifications. Sometimes the intensity of the stretch is decreased, sometimes it is increased. If the effect is not stated, it is because the accompanying photo shows the result. Even if you are working on the completed pose try the variations. I guarantee that they'll teach you something new.

Aids illustrate the use of a prop to help you do the pose with proper alignment; sometimes they provide a lever for stretching or protect parts of your body from overstretching. Sometimes the aids are simply for balance. Whatever their purpose, do not think of them as demeaning. In the most advanced yoga classes props are used freely. I work with them in every practice session.

There are many poses in the book that are not classical yoga postures; for example, many of the hamstring stretches. They are included because they are necessary steps in preparing your body to do the poses. You can't do what you can't do, so these stretches provide a way to get there. Besides, by doing these poses with attention to how you feel, they become yoga. Doing anything with attention to how you feel is doing yoga.

A note concerning the names of the poses. The Sanskrit names above the main heading for each pose are used internationally and are the original names. For convenience, however, English substitutes are also used here. Sometimes the names are descriptive and sometimes they're a direct translation. It's really not important what you call them; it's important that you do them.

For you own yoga program you can proceed in one of two ways. Either follow Chapter 21, "Basic Practice

Guide" or work progressively through the corresponding poses (all the first poses, then all second poses, and so on) within each chapter. Either way, it will probably take you six months to a year to do the more difficult poses. Once you are at that level, you can use Chapter 22, "Core Program," as the basis of your regular practice. The last two chapters are primarily for runners and other athletes, and are important for injury prevention. Chapter 23, "Suggested Program for Before and After Running," contains a balanced stretching and strengthening routine for runners. Chapter 24, "Yoga and Sports," suggests poses for you to improve your performance and to counteract the imbalances that a particular sport promotes.

6
MORE THAN JUST BEGINNING

PRELIMINARIES

The anatomical information and basic poses presented in this chapter are the foundation of all that follows. Regardless of how flexible you may be, it's important that these fundamentals are understood from the beginning.

Squaring the Feet

Most people have some misalignment in their feet that needs attention, not only in yoga but when doing any kind of exercise. Because your feet are the base of your skeletal system it is important that they are placed correctly. (When the base is out of balance, everything above must compensate.) What you are looking for here is symmetry. When doing yoga or any other forms of exercise, square your feet. This means that the feet face directly forward, the toes are relaxed and spread wide, the weight is distributed evenly between the outer and inner edges of the feet, and lifted arches shape the feet and support the body. If your feet turn out or in, place them so they are straight forward. If you stand on the outer edges of your feet, press down on the joints under your big toes just enough so that the tops of your feet are level. If you have collapsed arches, place your feet straight forward and turn your knees out just enough to

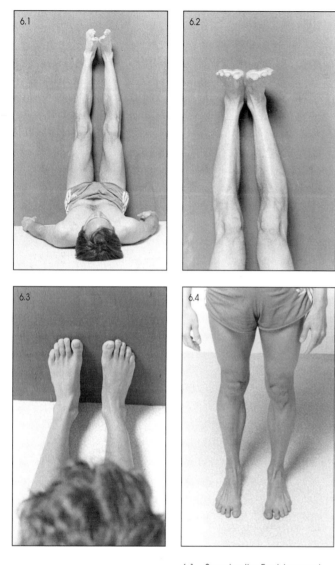

6.1   Squaring the Feet–incorrect
      position
6.2   Squaring the Feet–correct
      position
6.3   Squaring the Feet–seated
      at wall
6.4   Squaring the Feet–standing

lift the arches. The following exercise will help you better understand the squaring of the feet:

1. Placement. Sit sideways next to a wall. Now lie on your back so that your buttocks are against the wall and your legs are extended up the wall. Adjust your feet so that the soles are parallel to the ceiling. (If your knees bend, move two or three inches away from the wall, or far enough away so that you can comfortably straighten your legs.) Let the joints of your big toes touch and the heels be slightly apart.

2. Pose. Your feet will probably look like the photo, with the inner edges of the feet drawn down toward the body and the outer edges up toward the ceiling. To square the feet, press the inner edges of the feet up and draw down the outer edges until the soles of the feet are parallel to the ceiling.

3. Variation. Another way to practice squaring the feet is to sit on the floor with the feet pressing evenly into a wall. Keep the legs straight, with the kneecaps lifted. You can lean back on your hands. Squaring your feet is easiest to accomplish when you can see them, as in the sitting poses. Because you will not always be able to see your feet, become familiar with how squaring your feet feels so you will be able to apply the movement in all poses.

4. Variation. When standing, feel pressure on the ball joints under your big toes. Press here as you lift the arches of the feet. To line the knees up with the feet, contract the front thigh muscles and turn the knees to face directly forward. Learning to make these adjustments will take time; be patient with yourself.

Lifting the Kneecaps

The knee joint is to be treated with respect and care. Not only is it very complex because of crossing ligaments and vulnerable cartilage, but it also supports weight. In general, the knees are best protected when they are correctly aligned. The knees are aligned when each knee lines up directly with its respective foot. If the foot faces forward, the knee faces straight forward; if the foot turns, the knee turns. This is true whether the knee is straightened or bent, so always place your knees so each is directly over its respective foot. This sounds simple, but many of us habitually stand and move with a twist in the knee (most often caused by stiffness in the hip), so it takes careful attention to recognize and remedy this imbalance. To strengthen the knees, the quadriceps (thigh muscles) must be contracted when stretching the legs. Practice the following exercise:

1. Placement. Stand erect with your feet comfortably apart. Lean forward and place your thumbs above your kneecaps with your fingers wrapped around the backs of the knees. Do not bend your legs.

2. Pose. Contract your thigh muscles and draw the kneecaps up. Observe how the legs feel. This action elongates and strengthens the legs. Practice this often in the beginning. Once you understand the action, you can work without your thumbs above the knees.

In any pose where the legs are straight, the thigh muscles and kneecaps are contracted in this manner. The instruction frequently is, "Activate the legs" or "Lift the kneecaps." Remember: the correct action is to lift, not to push back on, the knee joints.

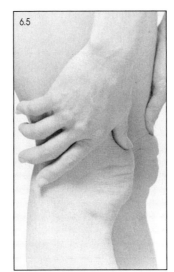 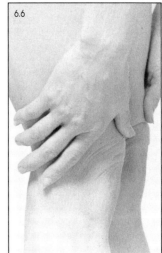

6.5 Lifting the Kneecaps–
     placement
6.6 Lifting the Kneecaps–pose

Activating the Thighs

Lifting the kneecaps in the manner just described automatically activates the quadriceps, the muscles on the fronts of the thighs. It is equally important, however, to activate the backs of the thighs. When you activate the thighs you strengthen and lengthen the legs. These movements, in combination with the positioning of the feet and knees as just described, allow the pelvis to assume a neutral position and the spine to elongate.

To activate the inner thighs, practice the following exercise:

1. Placement. Stand with your feet parallel and slightly apart, and place a thick book or wooden block between your thighs. Let the weight of the body go through the leg bones into the heels. Relax your abdomen. Lift your spine.

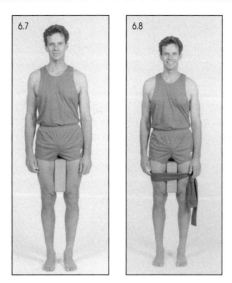

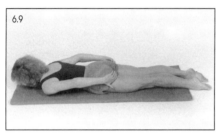

6.7 Activating the Thighs–block between thighs

6.8 Activating the Thighs–with block and strap

6.9 Activating the Thighs–lying prone on mat

2. Pose. Pause on an inhalation, and on an exhalation soften the throat and lift through the crown of the head. Pause on an inhalation and on an exhalation, with your quadriceps contracted, let your inner thighs lengthen along the length of the book. Do not contract your buttocks to do this action. It is important to isolate the movement in the legs. Keep going back and forth between releasing the spine upward and lengthening the inner thighs along the book.

3. Variation. Tie a strap firmly around the thighs while they are holding the book. Pause on an inhalation, and on an exhalation press outward on the strap. Practice this for a minute or two, and then vary it with the lengthening of the inner thighs described in #2.

To activate the upper hamstrings, practice the following exercise:

1. Placement. Lie face down on your mat or blanket. With the front of your chin on the mat, place your fingertips on your hamstrings at the tops of your thighs, right under your buttocks. Relax your legs and let them sink into the mat.

2. Pose. Now practice elongating and lifting one leg at a time. Even if you can't lift the leg, you will feel how the muscle under your fingertips tightens. You need to get familiar with how this feels in your legs so you can repeat it at will in other postures.

Pelvic Tilting

In all movement it is essential to preserve and nurture the four gentle curves of the back. (Reasons for this are explained in the section entitled "Elongating the Spine.") Because the pelvis is the base of the spine, the placement of the pelvis determines the curves of the back. Therefore, before you begin stretching, it is important that you get in touch with the muscles that move the pelvis. The following exercise will help you to do this. When practicing pelvic tilting be attentive to your lower back. Note how the alternate positions of the pelvis reverse the arch of the lower back.

To understand the placement of the pelvis, practice the following exercise:

1. Placement. Kneel down and place your knees so they are aligned under your hips and hips' width apart. Place your hands shoulders' width apart and directly beneath your shoulders. Check to see that your middle fingers point straight ahead. Lower your shoulders away from your ears, and stretch the back of your head and neck out of your shoulders. Elongate your spine.

2. Pose: Dog Tilt. On an inhalation lift your sitting bones and look forward (not up). Draw the chin in to lengthen the spine. Allow the back to arch slightly, the way a dog stretches after a nap.

3. Pose: Cat Tilt. On an exhalation contract your lower abdomen and draw your tailbone down. Drop your head and allow your back to hump up in the manner of an angry cat.

As you can see, the spine is longest when it is in a neutral position as illustrated by the placement position. When you lift the tailbone up, the back muscles contract and the abdomen stretches. When you draw the tailbone under, the muscles of the back elongate and stretch, and the abdominal muscles contract. Although these are effective stretches for the muscles along the spine, both of these positions do, in fact, distort the spine. By gently reversing these positions and feeling how the pelvis moves, you can become more familiar with that neutral (placement) position that is so important for spinal elongation. Remember that the spine is longest when there are no contractions on either the front or back of the torso and when the neck is elongated by lifting the top of the head away from the shoulders.

Elongating the Spine

The spine has four curves. The lower back and the neck are concave curves—they dip into the body. The tailbone area and rib cage are convex curves—they move out. For optimum health all four curves of the back should be preserved with no excess compression or curving in any segment of the spine.

A long, gentle S curve of the back ensures proper spacing between the bones of the back, the vertebrae. Proper spacing of the vertebrae is important because nerves branch out from the spinal cord between the bones of the back. If the curves become distorted, the

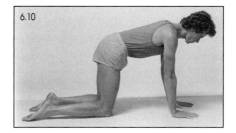

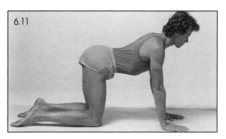

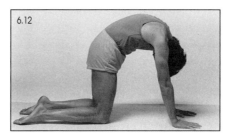

6.10 Pelvic Tilting–placement
6.11 Pelvic Tilting–Dog Tilt
6.12 Pelvic Tilting–Cat Tilt

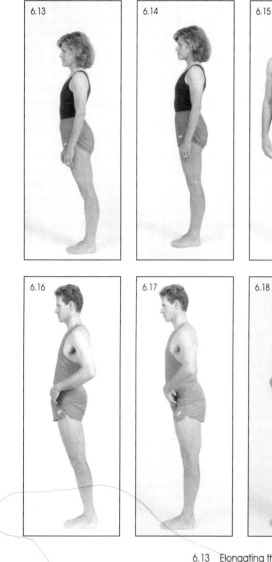

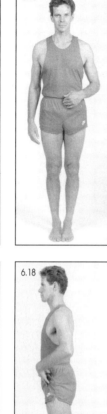

6.13 Elongating the Spine–incorrect position: weight forward

6.14 Elongating the Spine–correct position: weight over heels

6.15 Elongating the Spine–fingertips two inches below navel

6.16 Elongating the Spine–pelvis too far forward

6.17 Elongating the Spine–pelvis too far back

6.18 Elongating the Spine–pelvis over heels

spaces between the vertebrae are impacted. This may cause various problems to the vertebral column, particularly to the discs that are cartilage and susceptible to changing shape under pressure. The organs and structures innervated by the corresponding nerves may decline.

To understand elongating the spine, practice the following exercise:

1. Placement. Stand with your feet hips' width apart and parallel. Look down at your knees and make sure they are facing straight forward. Let the weight of your body sink down through your heels. Notice that when the weight is on the heels this places the hip sockets above the heels which enables the weight of the torso to go through the bones of the legs. Relax your abdomen. Align your shoulder girdle directly over your hips.

2. Pose. With your shoulders low, begin to gently press up through the crown of your head. On an inhalation, pause; on an exhalation, continue to lengthen through the crown of your head. Maintain the proper alignment of the feet and knees, and keep the legs active.

3. Variation. Do #1 and #2, and place your hands on the spot two inches below your navel. From this spot the pubic bone moves down. From this spot the torso moves up. Practice as in #2, but on each exhalation gently move the pubic bone down and the front of the torso up from this spot.

4. Variation. Place your fingertips at the front of each groin. When your weight is correctly placed over your heels there are very gentle creases in the groins and the flesh under your fingertips feels toned, firm. Move your hips forward (notice how your weight moves toward the balls of your feet) and feel how the creases at your groins disappear and the flesh under your fingertips feels hard. Then move your hips way back, more in a swayback position, and feel how the flesh at the groins gets flabby, too soft. After experimenting with the hips too far forward and too far back, find the middle position, with the flesh toned under your fingertips.

5. Variation. Stand sideways to a full-length mirror and experiment with #1 through #4. You will then be able to observe how these poses foster four long, gentle curves in your back. Sometimes seeing really is believing.

Aligning the Shoulders

Shoulders carry a lot of tension. They tend to be drawn up toward the ears or slouched forward or both. (A lot of this is due to sitting back on your tailbone. This causes the chest to collapse, and then the shoulders slouch as the arms reach forward. If you sit forward on your sitting bones the entire torso is forward, and the shoulders can remain low while your arms comfortably drop down to work, writing or typing or sewing.) As you may have noticed from the previous instructions, alignment lies in the middle, in balance. Aligned shoulders are neither dropped forward nor are they drawn back in a military "square shoulder" stance. Aligned shoulders are level and low, away from the ears. Viewed from the side they line up with the ears, and the shoulder blades lie gracefully flat against the rib cage. To align your shoulders do the poses that follow:

Aligning the Shoulders I

1. Placement. Standing with the spine long, move one shoulder at a time forward, roll it way up to the ear, turn the palm out, and draw the entire shoulder blade down the back as you lower the shoulder.

2. Pose. Turn both palms out and roll the flesh of the upper arms out. Feel how this flattens the shoulder blades against the rib cage. Notice too how this lowers the shoulders. Broaden the collarbones. Finally, let your arms rest at your sides. Moving slowly, practice this frequently during a yoga session and many times during the day.

3. Variation. Ask a partner to gently hold the flesh of one of your upper arms, right under your armpit. As you turn the palms out and lower the shoulder blades, have that person roll the flesh of the arm out. Be sure to stretch both arms, one at a time. If you have one shoulder higher than the other, it is useful to have this adjustment done more often to that shoulder.

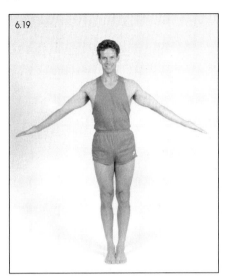

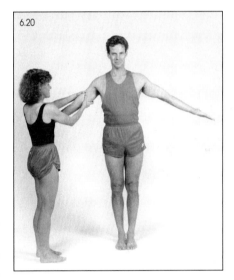

6.19 Aligning the Shoulders–arms turned out
6.20 Aligning the Shoulders–with partner turning arm out

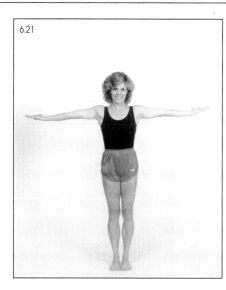

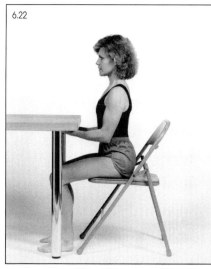

6.21 Aligning the Shoulders–arms to sides, palms up
6.22 Aligning the Shoulders–palms pressing table

Aligning the Shoulders II

1. Placement. Stand with your feet straight forward, with your legs activated, your abdomen relaxed, and your spine elongated. Lift your arms straight out to the sides until they are parallel to the ground. Stretch the hands out evenly away from the breastbone. Turn your palms up.

2. Pose. Pause on an inhalation, and on an exhalation roll the thumbs down toward the floor, simultaneously drawing the shoulder blades down the back. Repeat the movement up to ten times, and then, maintaining the position in the shoulders, slowly lower the arms. When the arms are down let the hands rest, and notice the position and the feelings in the shoulders.

Aligning the Shoulders III

1. Placement. Sit on a chair facing a table. Sit forward on your sitting bones so the weight of your torso goes through your pubic bone. Place both feet evenly on the floor or, if your feet don't reach, on books or a folded blanket. Put your hands on the underside of the table, shoulders' width apart, palms up. Draw your elbows in toward your waist.

2. Pose. Pause on an inhalation, and on an exhalation press your hands up into the tabletop as you simultaneously draw your shoulder blades down. Broaden your collarbones, and press up through the crown of your head. Continue for as many as ten breaths, and then, maintaining the position of your shoulders, slowly bring your hands to rest, palms up, on your thighs.

3. Variation. Once you get the knack of this, you can do this exercise without placing your hands under a table. Just bend your elbows forward, palms up, and do the action described in #2. Draw your shoulder blades down, broaden your collarbones, and press up through the crown of your head. Notice how the flesh of the front torso moves up, and the flesh of the back torso moves down.

Placement of the Head

A well-placed head is a sign of skeletal balance and gives a regal look. People whose heads are level are perceived as graceful and poised, maybe even "level-headed." Unfortunately most of us have slipped into less useful postures. For example, many Westerners, in an attempt to "get ahead" or perhaps to "stick their necks out," lead with their heads. These people collapse the backs of their necks, lift their chins, and carry the weight of their heads too far forward. Others are always "braced for the worst," with their chins pulled down and the backs of their necks overstretched. Still others may continually tilt their heads to one side or the other. This may be caused by cradling a phone against the ear or always carrying a briefcase or purse on one side. But whatever the cause, all of these and a million variations are indicative of skeletal imbalance.

A balanced head rests on a neck that is equally long from front to back and from side to side. The ears are level and, viewed from the side, the ears are in line with the center of the shoulder joints, the crown of the head is high, and the eyes' gaze is horizontal. To align the head:

1. Placement. Get a one-pound bag of rice off the kitchen shelf and stand in front of a mirror. Stand following the instructions for alignment given for the feet, knees, pelvis, and spine. Looking at yourself to see that your ears are level, place the bag of rice on the crown of your head. If you collapse the back of your neck, place the bag at the back edge of the crown of the head. If you stand with your chin pulled down, place the bag at the crown's front edge.

2. Pose. Pause on an inhalation, and on an exhalation lift right up into the bag. Let the throat be soft, with no effort in the neck, although you may feel some gentle stretching. Once you get the feel of this alignment, remove the bag and continue to breathe and press up into the crown. The head will feel as if it floats.

3. Variation. Once you have practiced in front of a mirror enough to get the feeling sense of this movement, try #2 without a mirror.

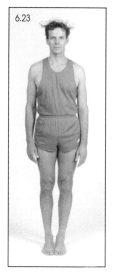

6.23

6.23 Placement of the Head–weight on head

A Word to the Wise

These alignments and directions are crucial to all the poses that follow, and incorporating them into other activities will bring positive results. But, there is one caution. While doing vigorous exercise, such as running, do not force your body into these alignments. Forcing your body into correct alignment before your tissue has adjusted to accommodate the change can cause great discomfort. For example, if your feet turn out, do not insist that every footfall of your next run be straight forward. You can keep in mind or visualize that eventually you will run with your feet straight, but do not suddenly change a pattern that is in every bone, ligament, and fiber of your musculoskeletal system. Practice these alignments in all yoga poses and any type of calisthenics, but not in any type of bouncing exercise. The speed with which you are moving does not allow the muscles, ligaments, and tendons to adjust to this new position of the bones. This can cause discomfort and possible injury.

If you are regular in your practice and careful about these preliminaries, the alignments will just slip into your body. Sometimes it happens so gradually and so naturally you may be unaware of the difference until someone notes it, or after a while you realize your feet are straightening. The body will not and cannot be rushed. Anyhow, the journey is the point, not the result. And, paradoxically, the more you are involved in the journey, the more easily the results come. Conversely, the more you work for results the more elusive they become.

7
SELF–RELIANCE

THE STANDING POSES

The standing poses are extremely important for maintaining the health of your back. Always position your pelvis so that your spine has four gentle curves (see Chapter 6). Maintaining length in the spine during these poses strengthens the muscles that support proper posture. The instructions for the poses will tell you how to do this. Keep in mind that you may need to modify the poses according to your body's needs, by experimenting with the aids and variations until you discover what feels best for you.

Standing poses also stretch and strengthen the legs. For athletes, learning these poses will improve posture and increase mobility in the hip, knee, and ankle joints.

All standing poses begin in Mountain Pose (Tadasana), even if the final stage of the pose is done with the legs apart. To start with Mountain Pose means that the standing pose is begun with the body in proper alignment. To get from Mountain Pose to a split-leg stance, jump your feet apart the prescribed distance. Jumping separates the legs with balanced movement.

•**Jumping.** To practice the correct way of jumping, first stand erect with your feet together. Inhale as you bend both knees, and bring your elbows to shoulder level with your middle fingers touching. Even

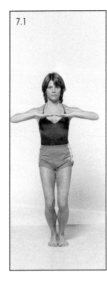

7.1

though your forearms are moving toward the center line of your body, don't collapse your chest. Exhale and jump your feet apart to the spread indicated for each pose. Make the jump low and silent, by landing on the balls of your feet and allowing your heels to descend with control. Check that your feet are still parallel and evenly placed, that is, your toes touch an imaginary line drawn from foot to foot. As you jump extend the arms straight out from the shoulders, palms down.

•**Turning the feet.** In many poses that follow, you will be instructed to turn one foot in and the other foot out. The reference point for this direction is the midline of the body. The heel of the foot that turns out (the front foot) is opposite the arch of the foot that turns in (the back foot). See illustration.

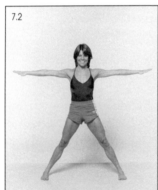

7.2

•**Centering the weight on the feet.** When practicing standing poses, ideally the weight on each foot is balanced over the center of the foot. You will soon learn how difficult this is—it requires your complete attention. To balance while doing any split-leg pose with your feet turned, bring more weight on the inside of your front foot and more weight on the outside of your back foot.

•**Protecting the knees.** To avoid injuring your knees, first lift your kneecaps, and then turn your feet. Keep your kneecaps lifted throughout the pose. Always keep your knees directly in line with your feet, even if your back hip moves forward. To avoid hyperextending your knees, stretch both the fronts and backs of the thighs, lifting your kneecaps high and not jamming your lower leg back. If you habitually hyperextend the knees, practice these poses with the weight at the front of the heels.

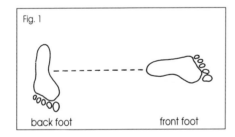

Fig. 1

back foot   front foot

7.1   Preparation for jumping
7.2   Completed jump

Fig. 1   Correct foot placement in
wide-leg standing poses

Caution: If you have problem knees, build your practice as follows.

Begin with leg lifts. Lie on your mat. Bend your left leg and place your left foot on the floor. Exhale as you raise your right leg, keeping your kneecap lifted and thigh muscles active. Keep your shoulders on the mat. Hold for five to ten seconds, breathing evenly. Practice to the opposite side.

You can practice leg lifts by sitting on a table with your thighs resting on the table top and lower legs hanging over the edge. Straighten one leg at a time, again lifting your kneecap and activating your thigh. Hold five to ten seconds, breathing evenly. Practice on each side ten times each day for two to four weeks. If you slouch while doing this, lean back on your hands to protect and elongate your spine.

Next, add straight-leg standing poses, for example, Triangle Pose (Utthita Trikonasana). Practice these four times a week for two to four months. Then add bent-leg standing poses, such as Warrior Pose II (Virabhadrasana II). Instructions for these standing poses are in this chapter.

Finally, proceed to Chair Pose (Utkatasana) at the wall, beginning with twenty-second holds, and increasing the time five seconds a week until you can hold the pose for one minute.

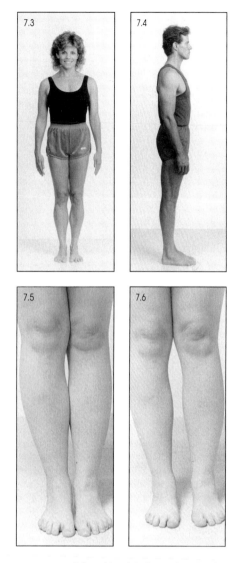

7.3 Mountain Pose–placement
7.4 Mountain Pose–side view
7.5 Knock knees–incorrect foot placement
7.6 Knock knees–correct foot placement

TADASANA

MOUNTAIN POSE

1. Placement. Stand with your legs straight, feet parallel, and big toes touching. Line up your knees to face directly forward. Make sure your hips and shoulders are level and your chin is parallel to the floor.

2. Pose. As you let your weight settle into your heels, lengthen your thighs and lift your kneecaps. Keep the pelvis in a neutral position, with the groin muscles soft. Do not grip your abdomen—remember, it is your legs that are your foundation. Lengthen your spine from your tailbone through the top of your head. Slightly lower your chin and keep your throat soft. Let your shoulders drop away from your ears, with your arms hanging loosely at your sides. Press up through the crown of the head. Hold for ten to twenty seconds, breathing evenly.

3. Variation. Draw an imaginary line down the midline of your body. Use this line to determine if your weight is evenly distributed on both sides of your body. Observe first the right foot, and then the left. Move up this center line and examine your entire body. Notice how just bringing your attention to the dull parts of your body affects the pose.

4. Variation. If you have knock knees, you will be unable to place your feet together without crossing your knees. In this case place the inner edges of the knees together and keep the feet apart, but parallel.

5. Aid. Stand with your head, shoulders, and buttocks against a wall. Observe whether both sides of the body touch the wall in exactly the same way.

6. Aid. Lie on your mat with your torso in a straight line. Square your feet and extend through your heels. Notice how your thighs automatically contract. Elongate your spine by lengthening the back of your head and neck away from your shoulders without tucking your chin. Move your shoulder blades and shoulders gently away from your ears. Place your palms down and lengthen your fingers toward your feet. Check that your neck and face remain relaxed throughout the pose.

7. Aid. Practicing Mountain Pose facing a full-length mirror gives you the opportunity to see your body in the pose and to make adjustments. Are your knees pointing directly forward? Is one shoulder higher than the other? Is your head tilted to one side? Where else do you need to bring your attention?

Benefits: Mountain Pose (Tadasana) is the foundation for all poses. It aligns the body, stretches the legs, and steadies the breath.

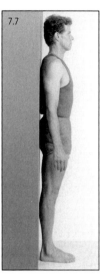

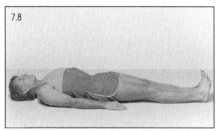

7.7   Mountain Pose–against wall
7.8   Mountain Pose–on floor

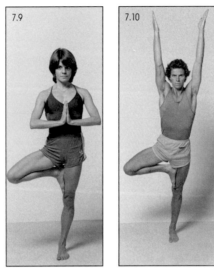

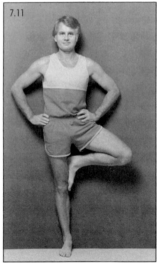

7.9   Tree Pose–hands in prayer
            position
7.10   Tree Pose–arms overhead
7.11   Tree Pose–back against wall

VRKSASANA

TREE POSE

1. Placement. Stand in Mountain Pose. Turn your right foot out, and place your right heel at the arch of your left foot. As you exhale, bend your right knee, and take hold of your right ankle with your right hand. Place your right foot as high as possible on the inner thigh of your standing leg. Maintain Mountain Pose with your standing leg.

2. Pose. Press your palms together in *namaste*, or prayer, position. Broaden your collarbones to keep your chest open. Press your raised foot and thigh firmly together, and balance your weight evenly on the inner and outer edge of your standing foot. Your bent knee will eventually move to the side as your hips and groins open. Lift through the crown of your head, and keep your eyes and throat soft. Hold for ten to twenty seconds, breathing evenly. Release and come back to Mountain Pose. Practice on the opposite side.

3. Variation. Stretch your arms up; keep your shoulders down. If you are tight in your groins or inner thighs, bending your knee may cause your spine to become swaybacked. To prevent undue curvature and therefore pressure on the lower back, you can place the raised foot lower on the supporting leg, and move the bent knee forward enough so that the front hipbones are parallel.

4. Aid. If you are having difficulty with balance, stand against a wall. Place your hands on your hips to judge whether your hips are level. Practicing against the wall will help you to feel more stable. As you gain confidence try Tree Pose again in the center of the room.

Benefits: Tree Pose (Vrksasana) opens the hips, groins, and chest, and steadies the nerves.

UTTHITA TRIKONASANA

TRIANGLE POSE

1. Placement. Stand in Mountain Pose. On an exhalation jump to separate your feet approximately three to three and one-half feet (or the length of one of your legs). Turn your left foot in 30 degrees and your right foot out 90 degrees. Keep your right heel in line with the arch of your left foot. Align your right knee over your right foot. Keep your kneecaps lifted and your front and back thighs active.

2. Pose. Exhale and move your pelvis toward the left as you extend your torso to the side and over your right leg. Place your right hand on your right shin or ankle, and stretch your left arm vertically overhead, palm forward. Turn your head to gaze softly at your left thumb. Hold ten to twenty seconds, breathing evenly. Release by coming back to standing. Turn your right foot in and left foot out, and practice on the opposite side. When you are done, jump your feet back to Mountain Pose.

3. Variation. Place your right hand on your right front groin to remind your body that in Triangle Pose you are to bend at the hips, not the waist. With your hand on your right groin, move your pelvis to the left as you come into the pose. As you extend over your right leg, place your right hand on your thigh or shin and lift your left arm up. Remember to keep your shoulders relaxed and away from your ears. Do not turn your head in this variation. Press out through the crown of the head.

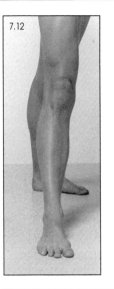

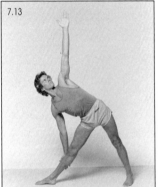

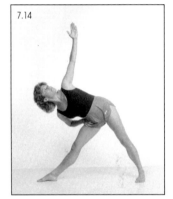

7.12 Triangle Pose–foot placement
7.13 Triangle Pose
7.14 Triangle Pose–hand in groin

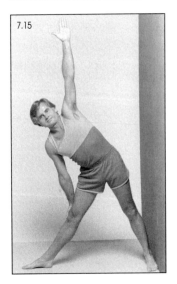

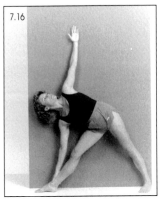

7.15   Triangle Pose–heel against wall
7.16   Triangle Pose–back against wall

4. Aid. Practice with your left heel against the wall and with your right foot turned out at a 90-degree angle. Practice the pose to both sides, as in #2. Pressing the outer heel into the wall helps to keep the back leg strong. Using the wall in this way develops confidence, balance, and strength.

5. Aid. Practice with your back against a wall to help keep your torso and legs in the same plane. Stand with your back to the wall and your legs apart. Place your left heel against the wall, with your right foot opposite your left arch and parallel to the wall. Bring more weight to the outside of the left foot and the inside of the right foot. Practice as in #2 or #3. Work to keep your right hip and shoulder blades on the wall. Do not force your left hip against the wall. Rather, use the contact of the wall to feel the outer right hip drawing back toward the left heel.

Benefits: Triangle Pose (Utthita Trikonasana) stretches and strengthens the feet, ankles, and knees. It also opens the hips and chest, and elongates the spine.

VIRABHADRASANA II

WARRIOR POSE II

1. Placement. Stand in Mountain Pose. On an exhalation jump to separate your feet approximately four to four and one-half feet. Turn your left foot in 30 degrees and your right foot out 90 degrees. Keep your right heel in line with the arch of your left foot. Keep your kneecaps lifted and your front and back thighs active.

2. Pose. Exhale while you maintain Mountain Pose with your torso, and bend your right knee until your thigh and calf form a right angle. As you descend turn your head to gaze at your right hand. Draw an imaginary line down the front of the body and balance your position on either side of that line. Take your left shoulder back slightly to open your chest. Lengthen your back leg from your buttock to your heel. Keep your left front groin moving back and slightly downward. Hold for ten to twenty seconds, breathing evenly. Release by coming back to standing. Turn your right foot in and left foot out, and practice to the opposite side. When you are done, jump your feet back to Mountain Pose.

3. Variation. In the beginning you may not be ready to take such a wide stride or bend the knee to a right angle. Practice with a shorter stride until the inner thighs lengthen and the hips open, but remember to always keep the front knee directly over the front heel. If you find that you tire quickly, you can practice with your hands on your waist until your strength and stamina increase.

4. Aid. Stand with your back against a wall, and with your left heel touching the wall. Move into Warrior Pose II following the directions in #2. Use the wall to help you maintain your Mountain Pose awareness, keeping your arms, shoulderblades, and right buttock in contact with the wall. Check to see that your right knee is directly over your foot and that your right thighbone is parallel with the wall. Allow your left hip to come forward if necessary.

Benefits: Warrior Pose II (Virabhadrasana II) strengthens the back and legs, develops strength and stamina, and gives an intense stretch to the groins.

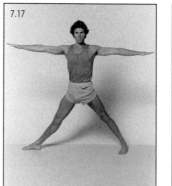
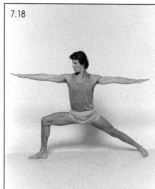
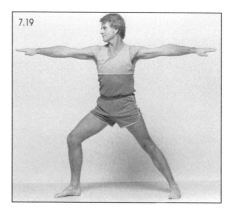
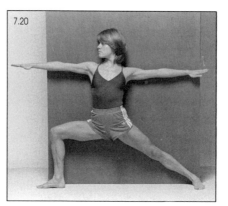

7.17   Warrior Pose II–placement
7.18   Warrior Pose II
7.19   Warrior Pose II–narrow
        stance
7.20   Warrior Pose II–back against
        wall

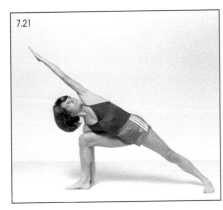

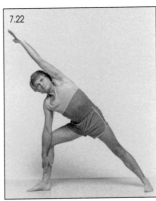

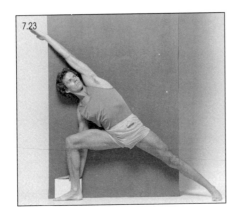

7.21   Side Angle Pose
7.22   Side Angle Pose–narrow
        stance
7.23   Side Angle Pose–back
        against wall

UTTHITA PARSVAKONASANA

SIDE ANGLE POSE

1. Placement. Stand in Mountain Pose. On an exhalation jump to separate your feet approximately four to four and one-half feet (or so your feet line up under your wrists). Turn your left foot in 30 degrees and your right foot out 90 degrees. Check that your right heel is in line with the arch of your back foot. Keep your kneecaps lifted and your front and back thighs active.

2. Pose. On an exhalation bend your right knee until your thigh and calf form a right angle. Check to see that your knee is directly over your heel. Exhale and stretch the right side of your body from your right hip as you extend your torso along your right thigh. Place your right fingertips or palm on the floor to the outside of your right foot, and extend your left arm overhead in line with your left leg. Turn from your hips to face the ceiling. Keep your face and throat relaxed and your gaze soft. Hold for ten to twenty seconds, breathing evenly. Release by coming back to standing. Turn your right foot in and left foot out, and practice on the opposite side. When you are done, jump your feet back to Mountain Pose.

3. Variation. Taking your front leg to a right angle may be difficult in the beginning, so narrow your stance to three and one-half feet wide. Bend your right leg so that your lower leg is at a right angle to the floor. Hold the inside of your right lower leg with your right hand. Press your right arm against your leg and open your chest. Keep your back leg active, lengthening from your buttock through your heel.

4. Aid. Stand as in #1 with your back against a wall and your left heel touching the wall. Place two thick books (or more, if necessary) to the outside of your right foot. Move into Side Angle Pose following the directions in #2, placing your right palm (or fingertips) on the books.

Benefits: Side Angle Pose (Utthita Parsvakonasana) provides an intense stretch to both legs and to the sides of the body. It also opens the hips and stretches the groins.

PARSVOTTANASANA

INTENSE SIDE STRETCH POSE

1. Placement. Stand in Mountain Pose and bring your arms behind your back. Place your palms together in *namaste,* or prayer, position, and turn your hands so that your fingers point toward the ceiling. If you cannot bring your palms together, practice variation #3. Exhale, and with a jump separate feet approximately three to three and one-half feet (or the length of one of your legs) apart. Turn your left foot in 60 degrees and your right foot out 90 degrees. Bring your right heel in line with the arch of your back foot. Keep your kneecaps lifted and your front and back thighs active.

2. Pose. Inhale and lengthen through your entire spine, from your tailbone through the top of your head. Exhale and extend your torso forward from the hips. Lengthen the spine and draw the right hip back to bring the pelvis level. Place your chin on your shin. Keep both legs straight and active by working your thighs. Lift your sitting bones up. Hold for ten to twenty seconds, breathing evenly. Release by coming back to standing. Turn your right foot in and your left foot out, and practice on the opposite side. When you are done, jump your feet back to Mountain Pose, and release your hands from the prayer position.

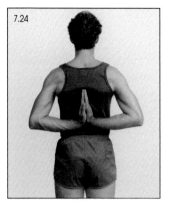

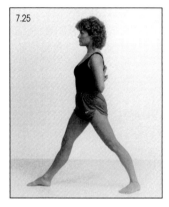

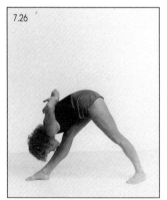

7.24   Intense Side Stretch
        Pose–hand position
7.25   Intense Side Stretch
        Pose–placement
7.26   Intense Side Stretch Pose

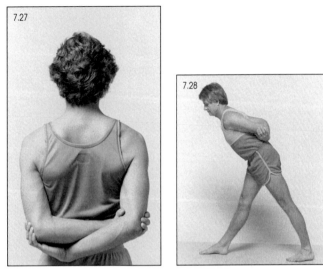

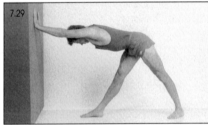

3. Variation. If it is not possible for you to practice with your hands in the prayer position, bend your arms behind you and take hold of your elbows, forearms or wrists. Practice as in #2. In the beginning you may also want to practice this variation: lower your torso to a right-angle position only. Keep your legs active. Remember to breathe!

4. Aid. Stand in Mountain Pose an arm's distance away from a ledge, table, or other piece of furniture that is approximately waist-level high. Step your left foot back three to three and one-half feet, and turn it in 60 degrees. Bend from your hips and bring your hands onto the ledge. (If you are using a table, you can place your forearms on the table.) Stretch through both arms and press your hands against the ledge. Keep your legs active by contracting your thigh muscles.

Benefits: Intense Side Stretch Pose (Parsvottanasana) is an excellent stretch for the entire body. In the upper body the shoulders and wrists become flexible, and in the lower body the legs and hips are stretched. This pose is excellent for runners and people who play racquet sports.

7.27 Intense Side Stretch Pose–holding elbows
7.28 Intense Side Stretch Pose-variation
7.29 Intense Side Stretch Pose–hands on wall

VIRABHADRASANA I

WARRIOR POSE I

1. Placement. Stand in Mountain Pose. Exhale and jump to separate your feet approximately four to four and one-half feet. Turn your left foot in 60 degrees and your right foot out 90 degrees, so that your right heel is in line with the arch of your back foot. Keep your kneecaps lifted and your front and back thighs active. Turn your palms up and lift your arms overhead. Exhale as you turn your torso to face right.

2. Pose. Exhale as you bend your right knee so your thigh and calf form a right angle. Remember to keep the knee over the foot; do not let the knee go beyond the foot. Activate the front thigh and back thigh of the left leg, as you extend from the left buttock through the left heel. Lengthen the front of the spine as you reach through the arms and the fingertips. Place your palms together. Keep your face and throat relaxed and your gaze soft. Hold for ten to twenty seconds, breathing evenly. Release by coming back to a standing position and facing forward. Turn your right foot in and your left foot out, and practice on the opposite side. When you are done, face forward and, as you lower your arms, jump your feet back to Mountain Pose.

3. Variation. If bending your knee to form a right angle causes discomfort in your lower back, or if you cannot turn your torso so your hips come level, narrow your stance and practice with your shin at a right angle to the floor. Be sure your breastbone (sternum) is aligned directly over your navel, not behind it, or your lower back will be compressed. If you have high blood pressure or if raising your arms overhead brings excessive tension to your shoulders, do not lift your arms overhead. Instead stretch your arms out to the sides or place your hands on your hips. Look straight ahead and descend your chin slightly.

4. Aid. Work with your back heel against a wall. Practicing with this aid will encourage your back leg to be active and teach you balance.

Benefits: Virabhadrasana I (Warrior Pose I) opens the chest and strengthens the shoulders and arms. It also strengthens the knees and stretches the ankles and calves.

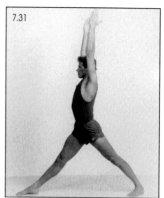
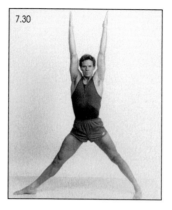
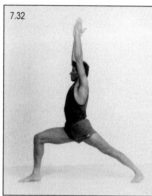
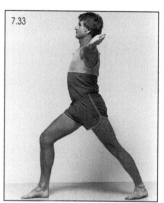
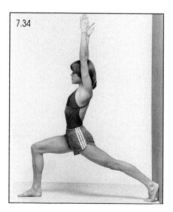

7.30 Warrior Pose I–placement
7.31 Warrior Pose I–torso turned
7.32 Warrior Pose I
7.33 Warrior Pose I–narrow stance
7.34 Warrior Pose I–heel against wall

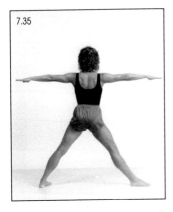

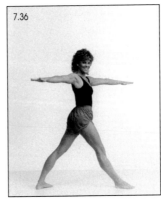

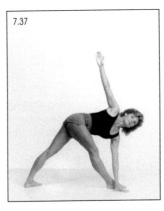

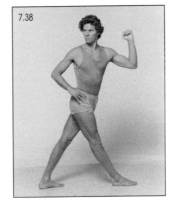

7.35 Revolved Triangle
Pose–placement
7.36 Revolved Triangle
Pose–torso turned
7.37 Revolved Triangle Pose
7.38 Revolved Triangle
Pose–torso rotation

PARIVRTTA TRIKONASANA

REVOLVED TRIANGLE POSE

1. Placement. Stand in Mountain Pose. On an exhalation jump to separate your feet three to three and one-half feet. Turn the left foot in 60 degrees and the right foot out 90 degrees. Bring your right heel in line with the arch of your back foot. Align your right knee with your right foot, making sure the center of your kneecap faces the same direction as your right foot. Keep your kneecaps lifted and your front and back thighs active. Extend your arms out at shoulder height.

2. Pose. Exhale as you rotate the left side of your torso around to the right. Bend from your hips and place your left hand on the floor near the outer edge of your right foot. Raise your right arm toward the ceiling. Keep your left leg active, and extend from your left buttock through your left heel. Lengthen your spine from your tailbone through the top of your head. Stretch your arms and shoulders away from your breastbone. Turn your head to look at your right thumb. Hold for ten to twenty seconds, breathing evenly. To release, come up from the hips and turn to face forward. Turn your right foot in and left foot out, and practice on the opposite side. When you are done, face forward, and, as you lower your arms, jump your feet back to Mountain Pose.

3. Variation. Practice as in #1. Before coming forward place your right hand on the right front groin. Bend your left arm, making a fist with your left hand. Raise your left elbow and, with an upward movement, swing your left elbow around to the right as you bend from your hips to come into the pose. This variation will give you the feeling of the movement that takes you into the pose. Repeat several times and then practice on the opposite side.

4. Aid. Stand with your back six inches from a wall. Position your feet as in #1, and place two (or more) books between the wall and your right foot. Exhale, swing your torso to the right, and place your hands on the wall, walking your fingers as far to the right as possible. Turn your head to the right. Keep your legs active as you bend from your hips, and place your left palm or fingertips on the books. (As you come into the pose, your right forearm will slide across the wall.) Look up at your right thumb, keeping your gaze soft. Breathe evenly as you lengthen your spine from your tailbone through the top of your head.

5. Aid. Place a chair against a wall. Practice as in #1, placing your right foot under the seat of the chair. Exhale and turn to face the chair. Step solidly on your left heel, and, bending from your hips, place your left hand on the seat of the chair. Drawing your right hip back, lift your right arm to the ceiling as you turn your torso to the right. Lengthen your spine, especially the right side, from your tailbone through the top of your head.

Benefits: Revolved Triangle Pose (Parivrtta Trikonasana) helps to relieve lower back discomfort. It strengthens and stretches the legs and increases flexibility in the hips.

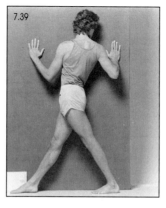

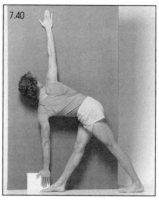

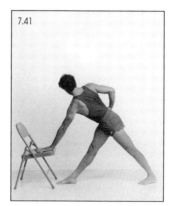

7.39   Revolved Triangle Pose–placement at wall
7.40   Revolved Triangle Pose–facing wall
7.41   Revolved Triangle Pose–using a chair

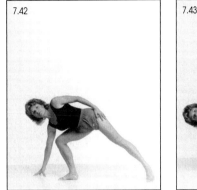

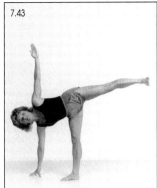

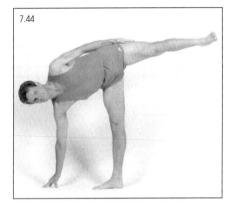

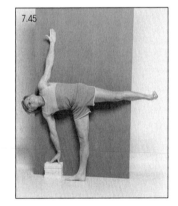

7.42   Half Moon Pose–placement
7.43   Half Moon Pose
7.44   Half Moon Pose–arm
       variation
7.45   Half Moon Pose–back
       against wall

ARDHA CHANDRASANA

HALF MOON POSE

1. Placement. Beginning with Mountain Pose, come into Triangle Pose. Bend your right knee and place your right palm or fingertips on the floor, approximately one foot in front of, and slightly to the right of, your right foot. Rest your left arm against your torso.

2. Pose. Exhale and shift your weight forward and onto your right foot. Make sure your right knee is in line with your right foot. Lift your left leg as your right leg straightens. Your left shin should be parallel to the floor. Keep both legs active. Extend from your left buttock through your left heel. Lift your left arm toward the ceiling, palm facing forward. Turn your head as in Triangle Pose and softly gaze at your left thumb. Hold for ten to fifteen seconds, breathing evenly. Exhale back to Triangle Pose. Release by coming up to standing. Turn your right foot in and left foot out, and practice on the opposite side. When you are done, jump your feet back to Mountain Pose.

3. Variation. Practice as in #2, but keep your left arm resting on your torso and your head facing forward. Turning the right thigh out, bring the right side of your torso forward and lengthen the right waist.

4. Aid. Place two books at a wall. Stand with your back close to a wall so that when you come into the pose the hip of your standing leg can rest on the wall. Practice as in #2, placing your fingertips on the books. Keep both legs active and lift your pelvis away from your standing leg and toward the ceiling.

Benefits: Half Moon Pose (Ardha Chandrasana) is excellent for stretching the groins and opening the hips. It strengthens the ankles, and lengthens and creates flexibility in the spine. This pose will help you develop balance.

VIRABHADRASANA III

WARRIOR POSE III

1. Placement. Begin with Mountain Pose. Come into Warrior Pose I to the right, palms facing each other. Exhale and extend your torso over your right thigh, stretching forward from your hips. Rest your torso lightly on your thigh.

2. Pose. Exhale as you lift your left leg and straighten your right leg. Your left leg remains straight and in line with your arms. Ideally the buttocks are level. Notice how your body forms a "table": your right leg is perpendicular to the floor, and your left leg, as well as your torso and arms, are parallel to the floor. Move your torso forward, as you stretch your left leg backward. Hold for several even breaths, gradually increasing the time to twenty seconds. Return to Warrior I and then come back to center. Turn your right foot in and your left foot out, and practice on the opposite side. When you are done, jump your feet back to Mountain Pose.

3. Variation. Begin in Warrior Pose I, with your arms extended out to the sides and at shoulder level. Proceed as in #2. Keep your gaze straight ahead and soft, and remember to breathe.

4. Aid. Use either a wall or a ledge to support the hands as you balance in the pose.

Benefits: Warrior Pose III (Virabhadrasana III) enables you to feel the dynamic qualities inherent in balance. It is especially recommended for runners for added energy and agility.

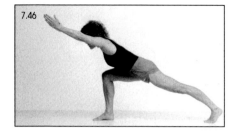

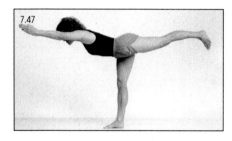

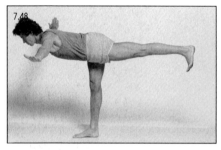

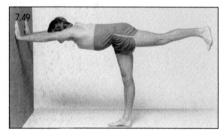

7.46   Warrior Pose III–placement
7.47   Warrior Pose III
7.48   Warrior Pose III-arm variation
7.49   Warrior Pose III-hands on
        wall

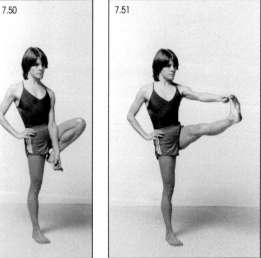

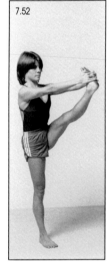

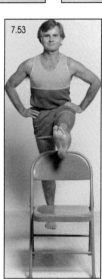

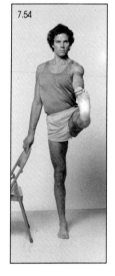

7.50 Extended Toe-to-Hand
Pose–placement
7.51 Extended Toe-to-Hand
Pose–with one hand
7.52 Extended Toe-to-Hand
Pose–using two hands
7.53 Extended Toe-to-Hand
Pose–with leg supported
7.54 Extended Toe-to-Hand
Pose–holding chair

UTTHITA HASTA PADANGUSTHASANA

EXTENDED TOE-TO-HAND POSE

1. Placement. Stand in Mountain Pose. Place your right hand on your right hip as you shift your weight onto your right foot. Inhale, bend your left knee, and lift your left thigh to your chest. Exhale and take hold of your left big toe with your thumb and next two fingers of your left hand.

2. Pose. Exhale and straighten your left leg, keeping your kneecaps lifted and your thighs active. Practice Mountain Pose with your standing leg and torso. Move your right hand to also take hold of your foot and stretch your leg higher. Hold for ten to fifteen seconds, breathing evenly. Release and come back to Mountain Pose. Practice on the opposite side.

3. Aid. Stand in Mountain Pose, facing a ledge, chair seat or back, or any piece of furniture onto which you can safely raise your leg. Lift your left heel onto the chair. Place your hands on your hips. With the left sitting bone moving down, keep both legs active, keep your chest open, and breathe.

4. Aid. Stand in Mountain Pose, with the right side of your body near the back of a chair. To help your balance and to help you gain confidence, practice as in #1, and place your right hand on the back of the chair.

Benefits: Extended Toe-to-Hand Pose (Utthita Hasta Padangusthasana) stretches and strengthens the legs, and teaches balance.

UTKATASANA

CHAIR POSE

1. Placement. Stand in Mountain Pose. Stretch your arms straight up with your palms facing each other.

2. Pose. On an exhalation bend your knees until your thighs form a right angle with your shins. Lean your torso forward until it forms a right angle with the thighs. Keep the arms stretching upward, encouraging the back of the torso to lengthen and broaden. Hold for a few breaths in the beginning, gradually increasing to twenty to thirty seconds. Release back to Mountain Pose.

3. Variation. Practice the pose with your feet four inches apart, and place your hands on your hips. As you bend your legs, be sure your knees are directly over your feet, not to the inside or outside. Vary your practice, sometimes keeping your heels on the floor, sometimes letting your heels come off the floor so you can bring your thighs lower.

4. Aid. Stand in Mountain Pose with your back against a wall. Bending at the hips, walk your feet out until your thighbones are parallel to the floor. Place your shins so they are perpendicular to the floor, and your knees are directly above your heels. With your abdomen and throat relaxed, hold the pose as long as your breath is quiet. Build up your time gradually.

Caution: Students with knee injuries should refer to the beginning of this chapter.

Benefits: Chair Pose (Utkatasana) builds strength in the ankles and thighs, and aids the knees by adding more muscular support to the joints.

Notes on Practice

The importance of practicing the standing poses cannot be over-emphasized. They prepare the body for all other yoga poses by developing spinal elongation and building overall strength of the body. They also bring flexibility to the legs. An excellent way for a beginner to proceed would be to spend the first six months to a year focusing mainly on the poses in this chapter. To round out your practice do a variation of the Hero Pose (Chapter 8), a variation of Shoulderstand (Chapter 16), and Corpse Pose (Chapter 20).

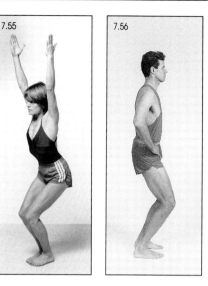

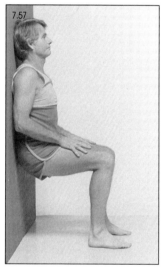

7.55 Chair Pose
7.56 Chair Pose–variation
7.57 Chair Pose–back against wall

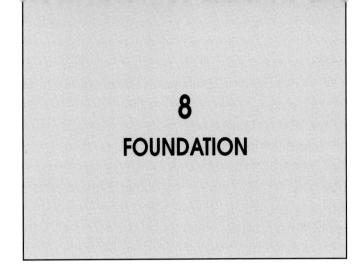

8
FOUNDATION

POSES FOR YOUR FEET, KNEES, AND LOWER LEGS

Because of the dictates of fashion, many of us—especially women—come to the end of the work day with sore feet. All too frequently we sacrifice foot comfort for styles of torturous extremes: high heels or pointed-toed shoes. We walk on hard, unyielding surfaces. And the tale of Cinderella has etched into our minds that somehow small, narrow feet are linked with beauty, benevolence, and queenliness. Large feet are reserved for the wicked stepsisters, who will always be denied true refinement and grace. Consequently we often cram our feet into shoes that are poorly designed and ill-suited to their task.

We have been sold an unhealthy bill of goods. The twenty-six bones of the feet need adequate space to distribute and balance the weight of the body. Lack of space leads to the overuse or underuse of certain bones, muscles, tendons, and ligaments. The result: the whole body must shift to accommodate its base.

Wear shoes that fit the size and shape of your feet. See to it that your shoes and socks allow space for your toes to spread. Every now and then cajole or pay someone to massage your feet. This kind person will earn your "footfelt" eternal gratitude.

Another way to bring health to the feet is to stretch them. When you exercise the feet you also

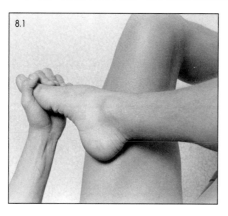

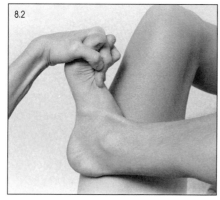

8.1   Fingers and Toes
       Entwined–placement
8.2   Fingers and Toes
       Entwined–stretching toes,
       sole, heel

involve your legs, knees, and hips. The arches of the feet are lifted by the muscles of the lower legs. Imbalance in these muscles can not only affect the arches of the feet, but influence the position of the ankles. Misalignment here necessitates a compensation by either the knees or the hips or both.

Most foot problems are mechanical. Proper movement may be the fastest, most effective remedy. Try all of the following poses, and work often, but gently, on the ones that reveal your greatest tightnesses. Practicing the variations of the Hero Pose (Virasana) will probably bring the most benefits. This pose brings balance to the feet and ankles, stretches the knees, and revitalizes the legs. Along with Shoulderstand (Sarvangasana, Chapter 16), Hero Pose is highly recommended for relief of fatigue in the legs.

FINGERS AND TOES ENTWINED

1. Placement. Sit on a chair or on the floor. Bend your right knee and place the side of your right foot on your left thigh. Interlace the fingers of your left hand with the toes of your right foot. Place the base of your fingers at the base of your toes.

2. Pose. To increase the stretch, extend through your right heel as you stretch your toes toward your right knee. Hold for ten to twenty seconds, breathing evenly. Practice on the opposite side.

3. Variation. If you can't get your fingers between your toes, place the heel of your right hand on the ball of your foot and wrap your fingers over the tops of your toes. Extend through your heel, and, pressing with your right hand, curl your toes toward your knee.

Benefits: The Fingers and Toes Entwined exercise spreads the toes and bones of the feet.

FOOT EXTENSION

1. Placement. Lie on your back on a mat. Bend your left knee and place your left foot on the floor. Bend your right knee into your chest. Then extend your right leg until it is almost straight, pressing your heel toward the ceiling. Relax your face, neck, arms, and abdomen.

2. Pose. Extend through your heel, and then through the ball of your foot, and then through your toes. Reverse the action by curling your toes back toward your knee and extending through the ball of your foot. Once again, extend through the heel. Roll your foot from position to position, repeating the full cycle three times with each leg. Then do these same movements to both sides with the raised leg at first at 60 degrees, and then at 30 degrees. Repeat the cycle with the raised leg straight.

Benefits: Foot Extension strengthens the arches, stretches the feet and ankles, and brings awareness to the feet.

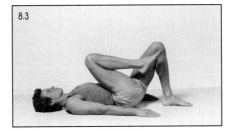

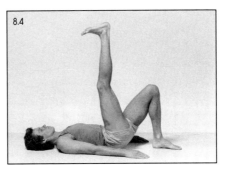

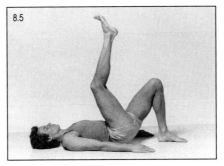

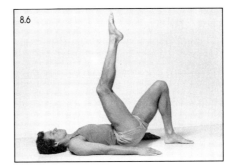

8.3 Foot Extension–placement
8.4 Foot Extension–with heel extended
8.5 Foot Extension–ball of foot extended
8.6 Foot Extension–toes pointed

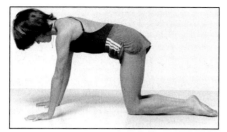

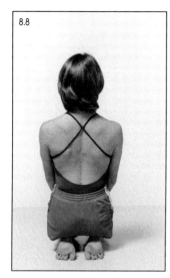

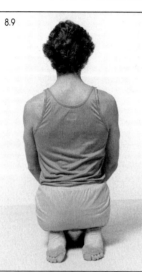

8.7 Diamond Pose–placement
8.8 Diamond Pose–sitting on heels
8.9 Diamond Pose–feet separated but parallel

The next four poses make up a series of stretches that are excellent for the feet and legs. Study and practice them individually first. The following photos show the complete series as it should be done. After completing the series, do it again in reverse order. Repeat the series four times to warm up. Once your muscles are warmed up, hold each pose for ten to thirty seconds.

VAJRASANA
SQUAT SERIES POSE I: DIAMOND POSE

1. Placement. Begin on your hands and knees with the inner legs and feet together. Point your toes so the tops of your feet and ankles are on the floor.

2. Pose. Exhale and slowly walk your hands toward your knees as you sit back on your heels. Stretch the inner edges of your feet back, keeping contact between them. Sit upright, lengthening your spine from your tailbone through the crown of your head. Place your hands on your thighs. Hold for ten to twenty seconds, breathing evenly. Slowly increase your time in the pose to two minutes.

3. Variation. Most people can't do this pose with the heels together. If your heels come apart, go back to #1 and separate your feet but keep them parallel. Maintain this alignment as you again sit on your heels. Let the weight of your body stretch the front of your feet and ankles.

4. Aid. If you experience cramping in the feet or discomfort in the ankles, place a rolled towel or small cushion under the ankles. The cushion should be low enough to allow stretching, but high enough for support. If necessary, combine this aid with the aid in #5.

5. Aid. If your knees are tight and your buttocks do not touch your heels, place a folded blanket or cushion under your buttocks (and on top of your heels). You may need more than one cushion, so experiment with different heights until you find a position that is comfortable. This aid will help to protect your knees from overstretching.

6. Aid. If one or both of your knees hurt, take a rolled washcloth or a rope and place it behind your knee. As you sit back into the pose, hold the washcloth or rope right into the joint. This makes more space in the joint and can make the difference between effective and painful stretching.

Caution: Never hold a pose if you experience pain in your knees. Consult a qualified yoga teacher for advice on how to proceed.

Benefits: Diamond Pose (Vajrasana) brings balance to the feet and ankles. It also stretches the feet, ankles, lower legs, and knees.

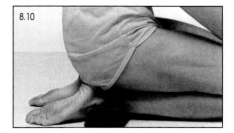

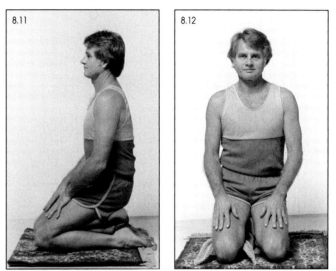

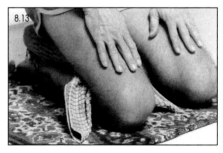

8.10 Diamond Pose–ankles supported
8.11 Diamond Pose–buttocks supported
8.12 Diamond Pose–roll behind knee
8.13 Diamond Pose–detail of roll behind knee

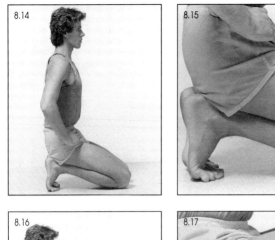

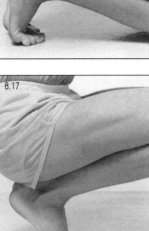

8.14   Kneeling Foot
         Stretch–placement
8.15   Kneeling Foot Stretch–detail
         of feet
8.16   Bent-Knee Foot Balance
8.17   Bent-Knee Foot
         Balance–detail of feet

SQUAT SERIES POSE II: KNEELING FOOT STRETCH

1. Placement. Begin in Diamond Pose, #1. Turn your toes under, using your hands, if necessary, to help turn your toes so all ten are on the floor. Keep your heels in line with your toes, that is, pointing straight up.

2. Pose. Sit on your heels. Be sure the lower back is long, with a gentle curve into the body. Now let the weight of your body settle into your feet. Hold for just a breath or two, and over time increase how long you hold the pose to one to two minutes.

Benefits: Kneeling Foot Stretch stretches the soles of the feet.

SQUAT SERIES POSE III: BENT-KNEE FOOT BALANCE

1. Placement. Begin in Kneeling Foot Stretch and raise your arms out in front of you at shoulder height.

2. Pose. Exhale and lift your knees from the floor until your thighs are parallel to the floor. Your buttocks remain on your heels. Hold and breathe evenly. Continue on to the next pose.

Benefits: Bent-Knee Foot Balance brings mobility to the feet and knees. Balancing poses teach poise.

SQUAT SERIES POSE IV: SQUAT POSE

1. Placement. Continue from Bent-Knee Foot Balance.

2. Pose. Exhale and stretch your heels back to the floor. Bring your knees as far forward as possible to stretch the Achilles tendons. Your back may round slightly to facilitate balance. Hold for ten to twenty seconds, breathing evenly.

3. Variation. Stand with the feet under the hips, and face a partner. You and your partner must both extend your arms forward from your shoulders and grasp the other person's wrists. It is important that you move together. Both of you must exhale, bend the knees, and come into the squat with the heels on the floor. Hold for ten to twenty seconds, breathing evenly. Stand to release. To increase the stretch, step farther away from each other and practice Squat Pose again.

4. Variation. Stand in Mountain Pose an arm's length away from a sink, windowsill, or the two knobs of an open door. Separate your feet so they are parallel and hips' width apart. Grasp the sink, windowsill, or doorknobs with both hands. Exhale and come into Squat Pose. Keep your heels on the floor. Hold for one minute, breathing evenly.

5. Variation. Stand with your back eight to twelve inches from a wall. Bend your knees and come into Squat Pose. Bend your elbows and press them back into the wall. Press your heels down and lengthen your spine. Broaden your collarbones to open the chest. Use your hands to press your thighs forward. Hold for ten to fifteen seconds, breathing evenly. Over time slowly increase how long you hold the pose.

Benefits: Squat Pose stretches the Achilles tendons, strengthens the fronts of the legs, and relieves tension in the lower back.

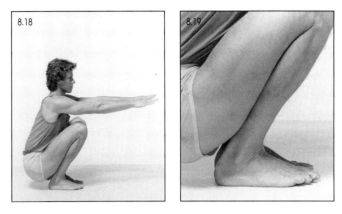

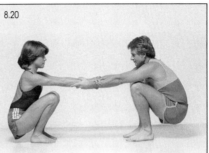

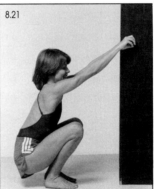

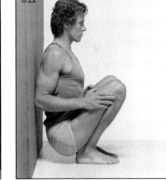

8.18   Squat Pose
8.19   Squat Pose–detail of feet
8.20   Squat Pose–with a partner
8.21   Squat Pose–holding
        doorknobs
8.22   Squat Pose–back against
        wall

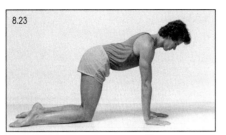

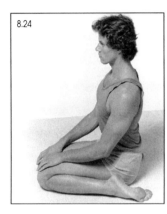

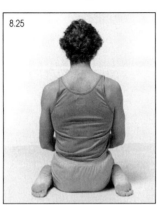

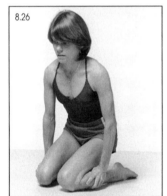

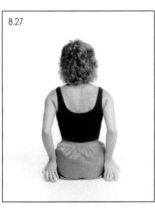

8.23 Hero Pose–placement
8.24 Hero Pose–side view
8.25 Hero Pose–back view
8.26 Hero Pose–rolling calves out
8.27 Hero Pose–palms on feet
8.28 Hero Pose–buttocks
   supported

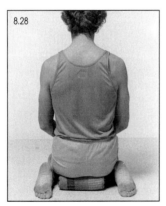

VIRASANA

HERO POSE

1. Placement. Kneel with your knees together and your feet separated enough to set your buttocks on the floor between them. Keep your feet parallel. Stretch the inner ankles and the feet straight back.

2. Pose. Exhale and lower your buttocks to the floor. Sit tall and place your hands on your thighs, close to your knees. Hold for fifteen to twenty seconds, breathing evenly. Slowly increase your time in the pose. To release, lean back on your fingertips. Straighten one leg at a time out in front of you, rolling the thighbone out and bringing the leg back down to the floor. When you are done, bring both legs together. If necessary, massage your knees with your hands to prepare yourself for standing.

3. Variation. Begin as in #1. Take hold of your calf muscles and roll them away from the midline of your body. Hold the muscles as you sit in #2. This variation moves the bulk of the muscles out of the way and allows the knee joints to open farther.

4. Variation. Once in the pose, turn the hands away from the midline of the body so the fingers point behind you. Place your palms on the soles of your feet. Press the little-toe sides of your feet toward the floor.

5. Aid. If you experience discomfort in your knees in Hero Pose or if the stretch on your thighs is too intense, sit on a folded blanket, mat, or cushion. The amount of lift under the buttocks should be determined by how you feel. You should feel stretch in the knees, but never pain.

6. Aid. As in Diamond Pose, use a rolled washcloth or rope behind the knee joint to relieve pressure. You can practice with this aid in combination with #5.

Benefits: Hero Pose (Virasana) balances the feet. It also relieves fatigue in the legs and is therapeutic for the hips, knees, and feet.

SUPTA VIRASANA

RECLINING HERO POSE

1. Placement. If possible, sit in Hero Pose, with your buttocks on the floor between your feet. (If this is not possible, continue practicing Hero Pose, using a variation or an aid.)

2. Pose. Exhale and lean back and support yourself on your hands. Slowly lower yourself onto both your elbows and your forearms. As you feel ready, drop your head back so that the top of your head rests on the floor. Then lower your chin toward your chest and rest your upper back on the floor. Extend your arms overhead with the palms up. Keep your knees together. On an exhalation stretch your arms and press your shins into the floor. Hold for several breaths, and over time gradually increase how long you hold the pose. To release, come up onto your elbows. Press your hands into the floor as you straighten your arms and come into Hero Pose. Release your legs.

3. Variation. In the beginning stay in the pose for a few breaths only and come up carefully. Allow your knees to separate, keeping the thighbones parallel and in line with your hips. Press your shins into the floor, and widen your abdomen.

4. Aid. If this pose causes discomfort in the lower back, use cushions or folded blankets to support the back. The blankets should be positioned just below the waist and extend to support the head. Have another towel or blanket folded under your head. Modify the height of the support according to your degree of flexibility.

Benefits: Reclining Hero Pose (Supta Virasana) stretches the psoas and aligns the feet, lower legs, and thighs. It also elongates the spine.

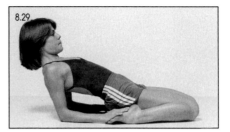

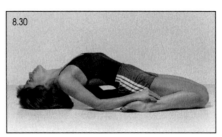

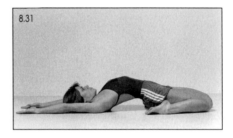

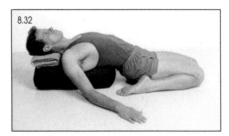

8.29   Reclining Hero Pose–
       entering pose on forearms
8.30   Reclining Hero Pose–
       head drops back
8.31   Reclining Hero Pose–arms
       overhead
8.32   Reclining Hero Pose–
       supported

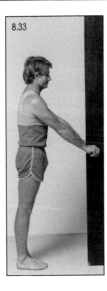

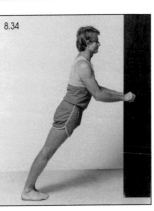

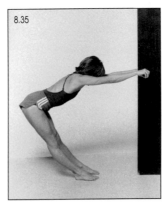

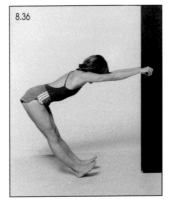

DOORKNOB STRETCH FOR ACHILLES AND CALVES

1. Placement. Stand in Mountain Pose, an arm's length from, and holding both knobs of, an open door. (You can also practice with your hands on a sink, a fence, or the open-window ledge of the passenger side of a car.) Keep the thighs active by lifting the kneecaps and elongating the legs.

2. Pose. Exhale, bend your elbows, and lean into the door. Keep your body straight from head to heels, which remain on the floor. Repeat ten times, holding for ten to fifteen seconds the last time.

3. Variation. To intensify the pose, continue holding the doorknobs. With the kneecaps lifted and the back long, exhale and bend at the hips. Stretch your buttocks away from your hands. Relax your neck and keep your head in line with your spine. Inhale, take a step forward, and come to a standing position. You can also practice by repeating #2 and then #3 several times, finishing in #3 and lifting the fronts of your feet off the floor so you are on your heels.

Benefits: Doorknob Stretch for Achilles and Calves stretches the Achilles tendons and calves, and lengthens the spine.

8.33 Doorknob Stretch for Achilles and Calves–placement
8.34 Doorknob Stretch for Achilles and Calves
8.35 Doorknob Stretch for Achilles and Calves–bending at hips
8.36 Doorknob Stretch for Achilles and Calves–on heels

ACHILLES TENDON AND CALF STRETCH

1. Placement. Stand in Mountain Pose, facing a wall. Place the right foot so the toes rest on the wall and the heel is on the floor. Step back three feet with the left foot; have the toes pointing directly forward. Place the hands on the wall at shoulder height and then straighten the arms. Lift your left heel and square your hips to the wall.

2. Pose. Press the left heel to the floor, keeping both kneecaps lifted. Place equal pressure on both hands. Hold for ten to fifteen seconds, breathing evenly. Come back to Mountain Pose, and practice on the opposite side.

3. Variation. To increase the stretch of the left calf, bend the right knee toward the wall. Keep your left kneecap lifted and your chest open. If you feel discomfort in your lower back, bend your elbows and move your torso forward so your shoulders are directly over your hips, not behind them. Lengthen the spine by lifting up through the crown of the head.

Benefits: Achilles Tendon and Calf Stretch is a marvelous stretch for calves, lower legs, and ankles.

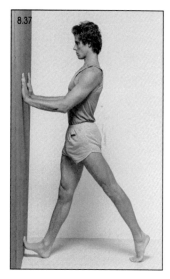

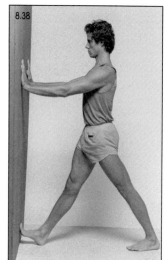

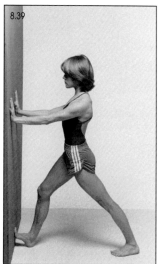

8.37   Achilles Tendon and
        Calf Stretch–placement
8.38   Achilles Tendon and
        Calf Stretch
8.39   Achilles Tendon and Calf
        Stretch–with knee bent

9
THE KEY TO POSTURE

HIPS AND THIGHS

The hip joint is formed where the pelvis and the thighbone (femur) meet. Its complexity is illustrated in the accompanying diagrams. Note that the muscles that surround the hip joint are connected to several places: the front of the spine, the hip bones, the sitting bones, the lower back, the thighbones, and the lower leg (below the knees). Underlying these muscles are smaller muscles and numerous ligaments that further stabilize the hip joint.

As stated earlier, the tilt of the pelvis determines the curves of the back. In turn, the tilt of the pelvis is determined by how the thighbones and the pelvis fit together. If the muscles, ligaments, or tendons that join the leg to the torso are too loose or too tight, they will affect how the pelvis rests on the thighbones.

If the muscles and ligaments around the hip joint are strong and flexible, the pelvic bones (these are the bones you rest your hands on when you put your hands on your hips) will be horizontal and symmetrical. Such balance in the pelvis ensures adequate space for the entire contents of the pelvic bowl, the viscera, and also decreases the chance of illness resulting from the stagnation of body fluids or the compression of nerves and organs.

This chapter contains poses for the front of the

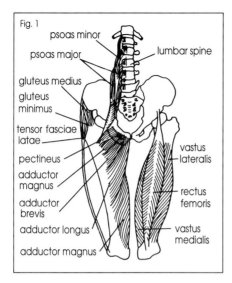

Fig. 1

- psoas minor
- psoas major
- lumbar spine
- gluteus medius
- gluteus minimus
- tensor fasciae latae
- pectineus
- adductor magnus
- adductor brevis
- adductor longus
- adductor magnus
- vastus lateralis
- rectus femoris
- vastus medialis

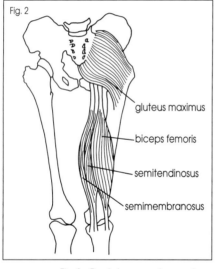

Fig. 2

- gluteus maximus
- biceps femoris
- semitendinosus
- semimembranosus

Fig. 1   Front view–muscles crossing hip joint

Fig. 2   Back view–buttock muscles and hamstrings crossing hip joint

hip (the groin area) and for the adductors, the inner thigh muscles that draw the legs together. There are a variety of muscles around the hip joint; many stretches for other muscles in this area are contained in other chapters. For a well-balanced pelvis it is particularly important to have flexible hamstrings (see Chapter 10).

A simple way to increase hip flexibility is to sit on the floor more often! The hip joint is capable of an enormous range of movement, none of which is encouraged by modern chairs. Just sitting crossed-legged rotates the thigh bones, stretches the inner thighs, and flexes the knees. So get out of the soft chair! If you are very tight, this position may be uncomfortable at first, so sit on the edge of firmly folded blankets or on a cushion. Sit this way regularly, and in no time you'll be comfortable on the floor.

Caution: The muscle that crosses the front of the hip, the quadriceps femoris, also crosses the knee. So does the fascia lata, the connective tissue at the side of the thigh. Move into and out of the following poses slowly to give yourself a chance to prevent any undue stretch to the knee. Anyone with a knee injury will tell you that it's not a very forgiving joint—it takes a long time to heal.

SUKHASANA

TAILOR POSE

1. Placement. Sit in Staff Pose (Chapter 17). Bend both of your legs and cross your ankles.

2. Pose. Exhale and bring the ankles in toward the groins. Use your hands to move the feet under the thighs so that the soles of the feet are in line with the outer thighs. Rest your hands on your knees. Do not collapse your lower back, but lift your spine on exhalation. Balance evenly on the front of your sitting bones. Keep your chin parallel to the floor and your eyes and throat soft. Hold for fifteen to twenty seconds, breathing evenly. Come back to Staff Pose and practice on the opposite side, reversing the fold of your legs.

3. Variation. Do #2, and stretch your arms overhead, interlocking your fingers. Exhale and press your palms to the ceiling. Hold for several breaths and return to Staff Pose. Practice on the opposite side, reversing the fold of your legs and the interlock of your fingers.

4. Aid. Sit in #2 with your sitting bones on the edge of a firmly folded blanket or on a cushion. (You may need more than one blanket if your hips are very tight.) Sit so you feel the weight of your body go through your pubic bone. Using a support will help you position the pelvis properly, enabling you to lift the spine.

Benefits: Tailor Pose (Sukhasana) opens the hips. It is a preparatory pose for more advanced sitting poses.

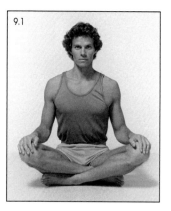

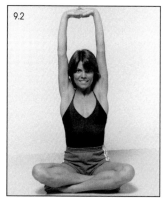

9.1   Tailor Pose
9.2   Tailor Pose–palms to ceiling

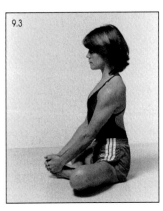

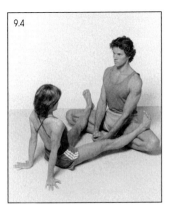

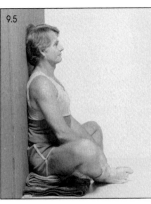

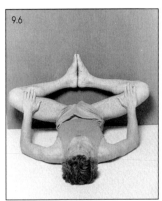

9.3   Bound Angle Pose
9.4   Bound Angle Pose—with
       partner
9.5   Bound Angle Pose—against
       wall with buttocks raised
9.6   Bound Angle Pose—lying with
       legs against wall

BADDHA KONASANA

BOUND ANGLE POSE

1. Placement. Sit in Staff Pose (Chapter 17). Bend your knees out to the sides and place the soles of your feet together. Draw the feet as close to the body as possible. Wrap your hands around the first four toes of each foot, one hand atop the other. Your little toes remain on the floor throughout. Remember to balance forward on your sitting bones as you lift and lengthen your spine.

2. Pose. In this pose it is often helpful to move with the breath. With each inhalation, pause; with each exhalation, lift your spine and allow your legs to drop closer to the floor. Do not force your knees toward the floor. Your legs will drop as the groin area stretches and releases. Hold for fifteen seconds, breathing evenly. Increase your time in the pose to two minutes or longer. To release, lean back on your fingertips. Straighten one leg at a time, rolling the thighbone out, and bringing the leg back down to the floor. When you are done, bring both legs together. If necessary, massage your knees with your hands to prepare yourself for standing.

3. Aid. Have a partner sit opposite you on the floor. Once in the pose, have your partner rest his or her legs on your thighs. The weight of your partner's legs on your thighs will help your groins to release and your legs to drop toward the floor. Breathe to lengthen the spine, breathe to soften the groins.

4. Aid. If your lower back collapses, sit on a firmly folded blanket or cushion. (You may need more than one.) You can also sit with your back against a wall for support, with or without the blanket or cushion. Without overarching the back, lengthen the front (anterior) spine.

5. Aid. Learn to lengthen your spine in this pose by using a wall. Lie in Staff Pose, with your legs stretching up a wall. Bend your knees out to the sides and bring the soles of your feet together as in #1. Using your hands, gently roll your thighbones toward the floor and press your thighs back toward the wall.

Benefits: Bound Angle Pose (Baddha Konasana) is excellent for the health of the pelvic region. It also stretches the inner legs and increases the mobility of hips.

AKARNA DHANURASANA

ARCHER POSE

1. Placement. Sit in Staff Pose (Chapter 17). Bend your right knee up and hold the ball of your foot with both hands. Sit tall and breathe!

2. Pose. Straighten your leg so your right foot is at eye level. Alternate between #1 and #2 so that your leg pumps. Practice ten times or so. Use a strap around the right foot if the hamstrings are tight.

3. Pose. When your leg feels warmed up, bend your knee and bring it back toward your right armpit. This movement stretches the hip and upper hamstrings. Keep lifting the spine. Alternate between #1 and #3. Practice five to ten times.

4. Pose. Begin with your knee under your right armpit as in #3. Place the right foot on the left forearm, cradled into the inner elbow. Place your right inner elbow around your right knee, and interlace your fingers. Keeping the right foot square and flat against the left arm, rock the leg from side to side. Stretch the hip; do not twist the knee.

Caution: If you experience pain in your knees, discontinue practice of this pose and consult a qualified teacher.

Benefits: Archer Pose (Akarna Dhanurasana) stretches the hamstrings, hips, and knees. It also strengthens the arms and back.

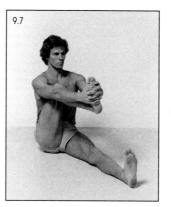

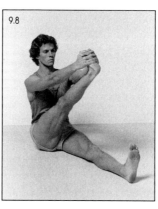

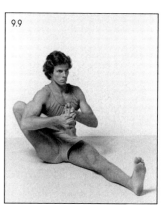

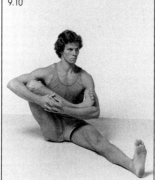

9.7   Archer Pose–placement
9.8   Archer Pose–straighten leg
9.9   Archer Pose–knee into
        armpit
9.10   Archer Pose–leg cradled

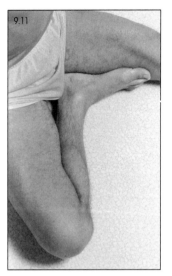

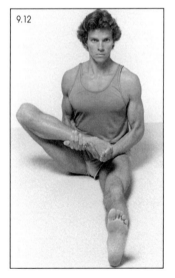
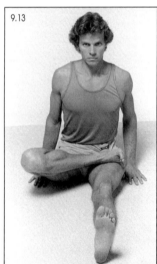

9.11   Half Lotus Pose–placement
9.12   Half Lotus Pose–lifting leg
9.13   Half Lotus Pose–foot on thigh

ARDHA PADMASANA

HALF LOTUS POSE

1. Placement. Sit with your legs extended in front of you. Bend your right knee and place your foot on the floor so that it is close to the right sitting bone. Let the right knee drop to the side, and press the sole of the foot against the inner left thigh. Look at the right foot and see that it is perpendicular to the right lower leg. Keep the foot in this position throughout. If this is not possible, place a folded piece of cloth under the right ankle and press out through the right heel.

2. Preparation. Cup your hands and, using them as a scoop, pick up your right ankle. Exhale, move the leg to the left and across the body. Do not change the position of the right foot; keep it squared.

3. Pose. Continue to hold your ankle and place your foot so that your heel is opposite your navel. Draw the heel as close as possible to the navel, and then bring the top of the foot to rest in the groin. Do not touch the right leg, and never press it toward the floor. Place your hands on the floor, sit tall, and let gravity lower your leg as it stretches. Hold for five to ten seconds, breathing evenly. Over time increase the length of your time in the pose to thirty seconds. Release by lifting your ankle off your thigh with both hands and placing your foot on the floor. Come back to Staff Pose and practice on the opposite side.

Caution: Never force the knees. If your knees hurt, discontinue the pose and consult a qualified yoga teacher.

Benefits: Half Lotus Pose (Ardha Padmasana) stretches the hips and knees, and strengthens the ankles and back.

STANDING GROIN STRETCH

1. Placement. Stand three feet from a table or another piece of furniture that is waist-level high. Stand in Mountain Pose, breathing evenly. Transfer your weight to your left foot and lift your right leg, placing the ball of your foot on the edge of the table. Place your hands on your hips to evaluate if they are level and equidistant from the table.

2. Pose. Exhale, bend your right knee, and lean forward. Keep the left heel down and the spine lengthening. Repeat ten times as a warmup, and then hold for ten to fifteen seconds, breathing evenly. Come back to Mountain Pose and practice to the opposite side.

Benefits: Standing Groin Stretch is a versatile groin stretch that can be done frequently.

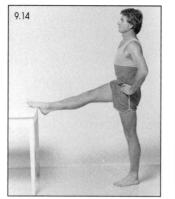

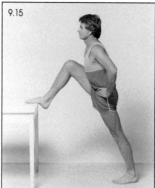

KNEELING GROIN STRETCH

1. Placement. Kneel and bring one leg forward to a 90-degree angle. (If you are more flexible, you can practice with your foot farther in front of the knee.) Interlace your fingers and place your palms on your front knee for stability.

2. Pose. Keeping the torso erect, exhale and increase the bend of the front knee. Do not allow this leg to go out to the side; keep it directly over the toes. Stretch through the back leg, keeping the knee directly facing the floor, not turned out. Hold for fifteen to twenty seconds, breathing evenly. Over time gradually increase your length of time in the pose. Release and practice on the opposite side.

3. Variation. To increase the stretch in the groins, lift the arms overhead, with the palms facing each other. Stretch up through the fingertips and keep the spine long. Slowly bend the front leg, keeping the knee directly over the toes. The Achilles tendon is stretched by keeping the heel of the front foot down.

Benefits: Kneeling Groin Stretch is an excellent stretch for the groins and upper thighs.

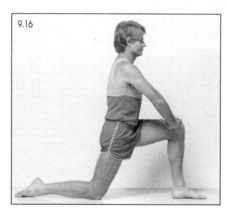

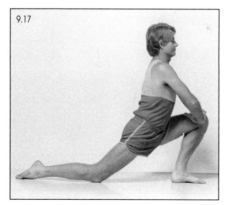

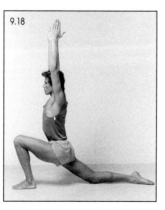

9.14 Standing Groin
Stretch–placement
9.15 Standing Groin Stretch
9.16 Kneeling Groin
Stretch–placement
9.17 Kneeling Groin Stretch
9.18 Kneeling Groin Stretch–arms
overhead

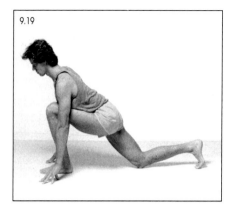

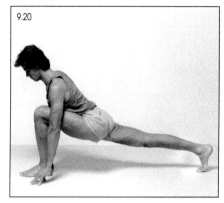

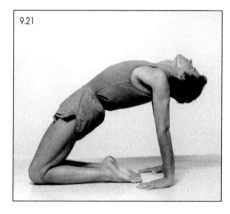

LUNGE POSITION

1. Placement. Begin by doing Kneeling Groin Stretch. Stretch your torso forward until it rests on your thigh. Place your fingers on the floor beside your foot. Turn the toes of your back foot under.

2. Pose. Straighten the back leg, keeping the kneecap lifted. Lengthen from the top of the head through the back heel. Hold for fifteen to twenty seconds, breathing evenly. Over time gradually increase your length of time in the pose. Release and practice on the opposite side.

Benefits: The Lunge Position stretches the groins, and strengthens the legs and back.

FRONT THIGH STRETCH

1. Placement. Sit on your heels in Diamond Pose (Chapter 8). Lean back slightly and place your hands on the floor so your fingers point forward. Keep the fingertips in line with the toes.

2. Pose. Exhale, lengthening the backs of your thighs and pressing your shins toward the floor, lift your buttocks from your heels. Your body is now in a slanted plank position. Keep your head in line with the torso or dropped back. Hold for ten to fifteen seconds, breathing evenly.

Caution: Do not do this pose if you have an injured neck. Do this pose very slowly so you don't strain your knees.

Benefits: Front Thigh Stretch stretches the knees, front thighs, and groins, and strengthens the back and neck.

9.19 Lunge Position–placement
9.20 Lunge Position
9.21 Front Thigh Stretch

NATARAJASANA

DANCER'S POSE

1. Placement. Stand in Mountain Pose, slightly more than arm's length from a table or another piece of furniture that is waist high. Transfer your weight to your right foot and bend your left leg, taking hold of the outside of your left ankle with your left hand. Stretch the right arm forward from the shoulder, with the palm of the hand down.

2. Pose. Exhale and bend from your hip joints, bringing your torso to a horizontal position as you stretch your right arm onto the table. Stretch from the left groin to the knee. Keep your body level and your left knee pointing directly back, not out to the side. Hold for fifteen to twenty seconds, breathing evenly. Release by coming back to Mountain Pose and practice to the opposite side.

3. Variation. Do #2, holding your torso in the horizontal position. Bring the heel as close to the buttock as possible. Be gentle. Hold for fifteen to twenty seconds, breathing evenly. Gradually increase your length of time in the pose.

Benefits: Dancer's Pose (Natarajasana) is an excellent stretch for the knees, thighs, and groins. It also strengthens the back.

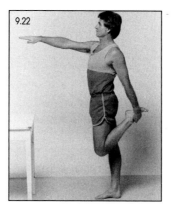

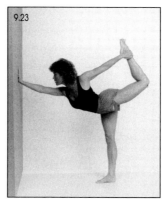

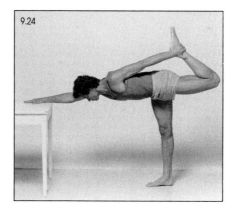

9.22 Dancer's Pose–placement
9.23 Dancer's Pose
9.24 Dancer's Pose–heel to
buttock

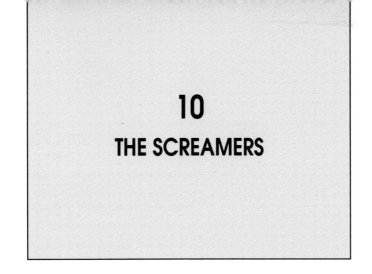

10
THE SCREAMERS

HAMSTRING STRETCHES

The hamstring muscles are aptly named. They contain a high portion of tendonous fiber; one hamstring, the semitendinosus, is fully one-half tendon. Tendons are far less resilient than muscles; like string, they are inherently resistant to stretching. This is why the hamstrings require consistent, patient work on the part of athletes and others who contract these muscles frequently.

The hamstrings cross two joints: the hips and the knees. Therefore the health of the hamstrings influences the health of both of these joints. Proper stretching of the hamstrings can increase the mobility of the knee, thereby relieving many knee complaints.

Excessive tightness in the hamstrings can affect the back, because these muscles are attached to the sitting bones of the pelvis. If the hamstrings are too tight, they pull the pelvis down and can cause misalignment in the back, the hips, or the knees. In short, the potentially negative effects of tight hamstrings can't be overemphasized.

Before proceeding to the stretches in this section, do the test for hamstring flexibility. The ability to raise your leg to a vertical position when lying on your back is normal (but not average). Even if you have normal flexibility, do some hamstring stretches; hamstrings are always tightening.

Besides stretching the hamstrings before and after every workout, or in a regular yoga practice, try to practice some of these poses throughout the day. The standing poses are most adaptable to this. You can do the Beginner's Hamstring Stretch easily. When on the phone place one foot on a chair and tilt the torso toward the leg. Or modify the Scissor Stretch by simply placing your leg on any support—a desk or table—and hold in that position. Regularity of practice will pay off.

If you have a back problem, you particularly need to stretch the hamstrings. The best way for you to stretch your legs is by doing the poses lying on your back. In this way the back is stabilized, and the legs must work instead of the back.

Caution: If you have a herniated disc, you can protect your lower back by rolling up a towel firmly until it is two inches high, and placing it crosswise under the lumbar. Be sure to bend at the hip socket so the stretch is felt in the hamstrings. Do not lift the leg so high that the lumbar is forced down into the floor, in which case the spine will suffer.

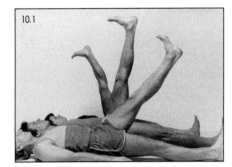

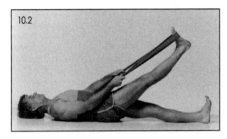

10.1 Test for Hamstring Flexibility
10.2 Test for Hamstring
     Flexibility–using a strap

TEST FOR HAMSTRING FLEXIBILITY

1. Placement. Lie on your back in Mountain Pose. If your chin is above your forehead, place a folded towel under your head so your chin is parallel to the floor.

2. Pose. Bend your right leg in toward your chest. Exhale and straighten that leg, keeping the kneecap lifted. Extend through your left leg. Keep both feet squared. Lower your chin slightly and relax your neck and arms. Lift your right leg as high as possible. The higher the leg, the more flexibility is present. Test your other leg.

3. Aid. If you have back problems, do this test by wrapping a strap or towel around the ball of the foot.

Hold the strap with both hands. Practice with a strap that is long enough so your head and shoulders remain on the floor.

Benefits: The hamstring flexibility test stabilizes the back, so the stretch comes entirely from the hamstrings. This test gives an indication of how often you need to stretch your hamstrings. The lower your leg is in this test the more you need to stretch; twice a day is the minimum recommended.

APANASANA

KNEE SQUEEZE

1. Placement. Lie on your back in Mountain Pose. If your chin is higher than your forehead, place a folded towel under your head. Bend your right knee in toward your chest. Interlace the fingers and hold the leg below the knee. (If you experience discomfort in your knee, hold behind the knee on the thigh.)

2. Pose. Exhale and squeeze your knee into your chest. Keep your left leg straight and active. Let your head and shoulders remain on the floor. Hold for up to twenty seconds, breathing evenly. Release to supine Mountain Pose and practice on the opposite side.

3. Variation. Do this pose standing. Begin in Mountain Pose. Bend your right knee and lift your right leg toward the chest. Interlace the fingers below the knee and squeeze the leg in toward your chest. Bring the knee to the torso, rather than lowering the torso to the knee. Keep your hipbones level. Hold for twenty seconds, breathing evenly. Release to Mountain Pose and practice on the opposite side. Stand with your back against the wall if balance is a problem.

Benefits: Knee Squeeze (Apanasana) stretches the hamstrings and groins.

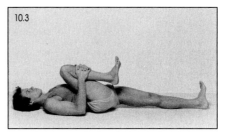

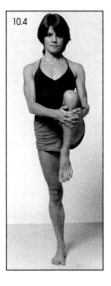

10.3   Knee Squeeze
10.4   Knee Squeeze–standing

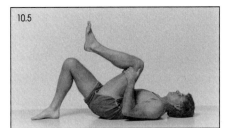

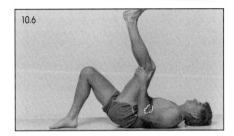

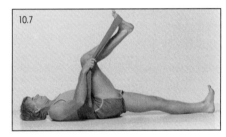

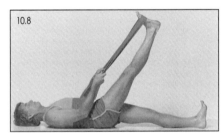

10.5 Beginner's Bent-Knee Hamstring Stretch–placement

10.6 Beginner's Bent-Knee Hamstring Stretch

10.7 Progressive Hamstring Stretch–placement

10.8 Progressive Hamstring Stretch

SUPTA PADANGUSTHASANA, VARIATION

BEGINNER'S BENT-KNEE HAMSTRING STRETCH

1. Placement. Lie on your back in Mountain Pose. If your chin is higher than your forehead, place a folded towel under your head. Bend your right leg and place your right foot on the floor. Bend the left knee toward the chest, gently holding behind the left knee with both hands.

2. Pose. Exhale and straighten the left leg as much as possible without lowering the knee. Extend the heel. Bend your leg and repeat the pose ten times, breathing evenly. Hold the last stretch for twenty seconds. Release to supine Mountain Pose and practice on the opposite side.

Benefits: Beginner's Bent-Knee Hamstring Stretch (Supta Padangusthasana, variation) supports the back as the hamstrings stretch.

SUPTA PADANGUSTHASANA, VARIATION

PROGRESSIVE HAMSTRING STRETCH

1. Placement. Lie on your back in Mountain Pose. If your chin is higher than your forehead, place a folded towel under your head. Bend your right leg in toward your chest and wrap a towel, tie, sock, or strap around the ball of your foot. Keep your left leg in Mountain Pose.

2. Pose. Exhale and extend through the heel as you straighten the right leg. Keep your elbows close to your torso and use the leverage of your arms to lift your leg higher. Do not push the back of your head into the floor. Hold at the highest point for fifteen to twenty seconds, breathing evenly. Release to supine Mountain Pose and practice on the opposite side.

Benefits: Progressive Hamstring Stretch (Supta Padangusthasana, variation) is an excellent way to stretch the hamstrings, calves, and Achilles tendons while protecting the back. When asked which hamstring stretch is the most effective, novice stretchers almost always choose this one.

SUPTA PADANGUSTHASANA

SUPINE HAND-TO-FOOT POSE

1. Placement. Lie on your back in Mountain Pose. If your chin is higher than your forehead, place a folded towel under your head. Bend your right knee in toward your chest, and grasp your big toe with the first two fingers and the thumb of the right hand. Keep your left leg straight and on the floor, and place your left hand on that thigh.

2. Pose. Exhale and lengthen through the heel as you straighten the right leg. Keep your right shoulder on the floor. Breathe evenly and hold for ten to fifteen seconds. Exhale and bend your right elbow out, and lift your head and upper torso toward your leg. The leg is stretched farther overhead as you bring your head to your knee. Hold for two or three breaths. Bring the head back to the floor. Bend your right knee, release your toe hold, and lower your leg to Mountain Pose. Practice on the opposite side.

3. Pose. After practicing #2, straighten your right leg toward the ceiling. Exhale and lower your leg out and down to the right. Turn your toes toward the floor and stretch the inside of your heel. Hold for ten to fifteen seconds, breathing evenly. Exhale and bring the leg back up and then lower it to Mountain Pose. Practice on the opposite side.

4. Aid. Have a partner press his or her palms down on your left hipbone to help you maintain balance in #3. Now gravity can be the lever while you give in to the stretch. Hold for fifteen seconds, breathing evenly.

Benefits: Supine Hand-to-Foot Pose (Supta Padangusthasana) stretches the legs, opens the hips, and strengthens the abdomen.

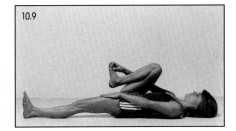

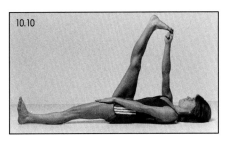

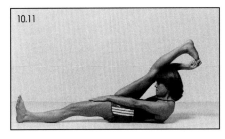

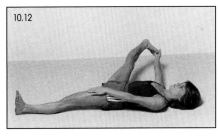

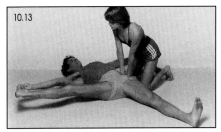

10.9   Supine Hand-to-Foot Pose—placement
10.10 Supine Hand-to-Foot Pose
10.11 Supine Hand-to-Foot Pose—head to leg
10.12 Supine Hand-to-Foot Pose—leg to side
10.13 Supine Hand-to-Foot Pose—with partner

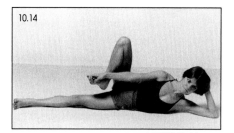

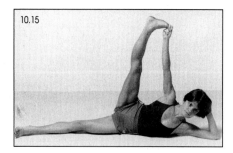

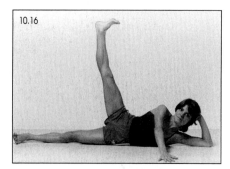

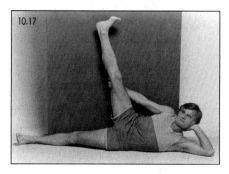

RECLINING SIDE STRETCH

1. Placement. Lie on your back in Mountain Pose. Roll onto your left side, and bend your left arm to support your head, with your left hand placed above your left ear. Keep your left arm in line with your extended, straight legs.

2. Pose. Exhale, bend your right leg, and grasp your right big toe with your right thumb and the next two fingers. Exhale and straighten your right leg. Keep the pelvic bones in a vertical plane. Keep both legs active. Hold for fifteen to twenty seconds, breathing evenly. Lower your leg and then your head, and roll over to your right side and repeat the pose.

3. Variation. Maintaining the stretch of the legs, the alignment of the body, and the balance is difficult in the beginning. Practice #1 with the right hand on the floor in front of the chest. Then do #2 without holding the toe.

4. Aid. Do the pose with your back to the wall, beginning in #1, with both buttocks one to two inches from the wall. Eventually work with both buttocks touching the wall. Hold the raised leg behind the thigh or with a belt around the foot.

Benefits: Reclining Side Stretch (Anantasana) stretches the hamstrings and helps to strengthen and stretch the pelvic area.

10.14 Reclining Side Stretch–placement
10.15 Reclining Side Stretch
10.16 Reclining Side Stretch–with arm support
10.17 Reclining Side Stretch–back against wall

UTTHITA HASTA PADANGUSTHASANA,
VARIATION

BEGINNER'S HAMSTRING STRETCH

1. Placement. Stand sideways and at arm's length from a chair that is placed against a wall, desk, or counter. Place your hands on your hips, and lift your right foot onto the seat or back of the chair. Straighten this leg and make sure your knee faces the ceiling. Keep your hips and shoulders level.

2. Pose. Exhale and, bending at the hip joint, tilt your torso laterally toward your raised leg. Keep both legs active and the kneecaps lifted. Hold for ten to fifteen seconds, breathing evenly. Exhale, lower your leg back to Mountain Pose. Practice on the opposite side. As your flexibility increases, practice with your leg on a higher prop.

3. Variation. Stretch the arm corresponding to your standing leg overhead, palm facing in.

Benefits: Beginner's Hamstring Stretch (Utthita Hasta Padangusthasana, variation) is a versatile stretch to do throughout the day. It stretches the hamstrings, Achilles tendons, and the sides of the body.

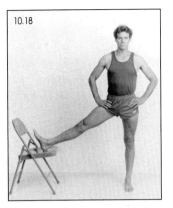
10.18

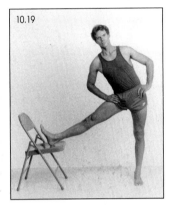
10.19

10.18 Beginner's Hamstring
        Stretch–placement
10.19 Beginner's Hamstring Stretch

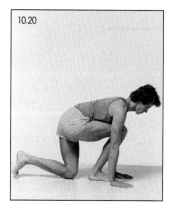

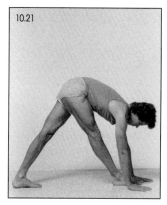

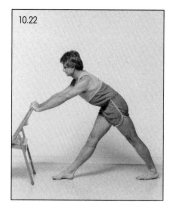

10.20 Runner's Warm-Up–
placement
10.21 Runner's Warm-Up
10.22 Runner's Warm-Up–with
chair

PARSVOTTANASANA, VARIATION

RUNNER'S WARM-UP

1. Placement. Begin on all fours: the hands are directly under the shoulders, and the knees are together. Place your right foot on the floor in line with your left knee and about four to six inches away. Turn the toes of the left foot under.

2. Pose. Exhale and slowly stand to straighten both legs, leaving your hands and torso stretched down toward the floor. Lift your buttocks up. To warm up your ankles, knees, and hips, slowly bend and then straighten your legs several times. Finally, hold with straight legs and the back heel down for ten to fifteen seconds, breathing evenly. Come back down on all fours and practice on the opposite side.

3. Aid. This pose may be very difficult in the beginning. To ease the stretch, place yourself in front of a chair, step or table. Place your feet as described in #1 and your hands on the chair seat. Now follow directions for #2. Be sure to relax your throat and abdomen.

Benefits: Runner's Warm-Up (Parsvottanasana, variation) warms up the ankles, knees, and hips, and stretches the legs.

UTTHITA HASTA PADANGUSTHASANA

SCISSOR STRETCH

1. Placement. Stand in Mountain Pose, approximately an arm's length away from the seat or back of a chair. Placing your hands on your hips, lift your right leg, and, depending on your flexibility, place your heel on the seat or back of a chair. Keep your hips level and your thighs active. Stretch your arms overhead and slightly behind your ears, palms facing in.

2. Pose. Keep your spine lengthened, and on an exhalation, move your torso toward your leg like scissors closing. Remember to bend from the hip joint. Keep both the front and the back of the torso long. At first you may not close very far. Hold at your maximum stretch for fifteen seconds, breathing evenly. To release, lift your arms and torso as a single unit. Lower your arms to your hips and bring your raised leg back to Mountain Pose. Practice on the opposite side.

3. Variation. Those who are more flexible and can keep the spine fully lengthened can take hold of the foot.

Benefits: Scissor Stretch (Utthita Hasta Padangusthasana) stretches the hamstrings and strengthens the back.

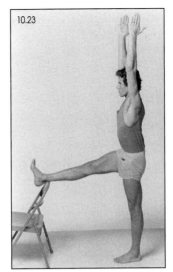
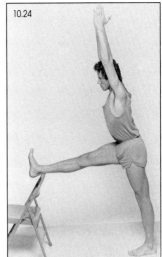
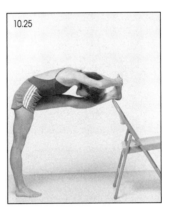

10.23   Scissor Stretch–placement
10.24   Scissor Stretch
10.25   Scissor Stretch–variation
        holding foot

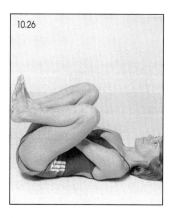

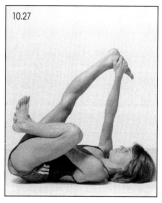

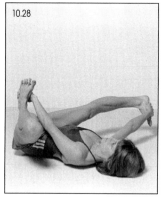

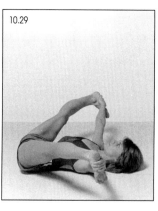

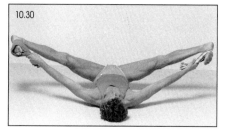

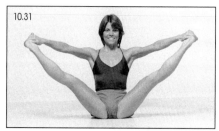

10.26 Butterfly Hamstring
Stretch–placement
10.27 With one leg straight
10.28 With leg to side
10.29 With both legs
10.30 With straps
10.31 Butterfly Hamstring
Stretch–seated

UPAVISTHA KONASANA, VARIATION

BUTTERFLY HAMSTRING STRETCH

1. Placement. Lie on your back in Mountain Pose. If your chin is higher than your forehead, place a folded towel under your head. Bend both knees into your chest. Turn the backs of your hands toward each other, and then hold each foot from the inner arch with the corresponding hand. Keep your shoulders and head on the floor.

2. Pose. Exhale and straighten your right leg to the ceiling. Hold at your maximum stretch for a full breath: an inhalation and an exhalation. Bend the right knee and then repeat with the left leg. Slowly repeat as many as twenty times with each leg, breathing evenly throughout. On the last movement hold for ten seconds on each side.

3. Pose. Exhale and let your knees drop out to the sides. Stretch your right leg as far to the right as possible. Hold at your maximum stretch for a full breath. Bring the right leg back to its original position. Now take your left leg to the far left. Slowly repeat as many as twenty times with each leg. On the last movement hold for ten seconds on each side.

4. Pose. Exhale and stretch both legs at the same time as far to the sides as possible. Hold at your maximum stretch for a full breath. Bend your legs back to their original position. Slowly increase your time to ten repetitions, holding the final movement for ten to fifteen seconds.

5. Aid. If you can't hold the feet and keep your shoulders and head on the floor, wrap a towel or strap around the balls of each foot, holding a towel or strap in each hand. Proceed as described in #2, #3, and #4.

6. Variation. Eventually this pose is done while balancing on the sitting bones. Don't be in any hurry to do this: it requires supple hamstrings and the back must be strong enough that you can sit without collapsing at the waist.

Benefits: Butterfly Hamstring Stretch (Upavistha Konasana, variation) stretches the hamstrings and adductors, and strengthens the hands and back.

11
SAVE THE PSOAS

STOMACH STRENGTHENERS

Leg Lifts strengthen the stomach and the lower back. But as anyone with a bad back knows, if these are done incorrectly or before the body is strong enough, Leg Lifts can cause painful backaches. Here's why.

Attached to the front side of the lumbar spine (the waist or lower back area) is the psoas (pronounced "so as") muscle, a muscle important to overall posture. It attaches to the anterior side of all five lumbar vertebrae, and then descends downward in the pelvis, crosses the hip joint, and connects to the inner edge of the thighbone. This muscle initiates walking and lifts the thighbone up.

The muscles that act in opposition to the psoas are the abdominals, the muscles that line the surface of the abdomen. For correct positioning of the pelvis, the psoas and abdominals should have equal tone, flexibility, and strength. One example of an imbalance between these sets of muscles can be observed in a person who has a sway back. As illustrated, in the swayback posture the abdominal muscles are lax and the psoas has to overwork to hold the body upright. The psoas, held in a state of semicontraction, then shortens. This pulls the lower back forward, overarching the spine and compressing the discs of the lower back. This spells misery!

You can see why runners may be prone to this

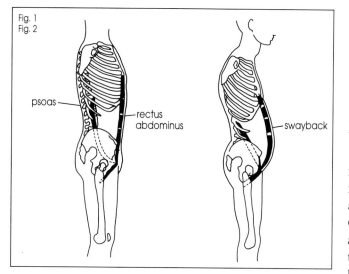

Fig. 1
Fig. 2

psoas — rectus abdominus

swayback

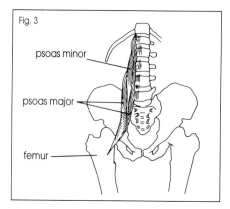

Fig. 3

psoas minor

psoas major

femur

Fig. 1   Balanced psoas and abdominals
Fig. 2   Imbalance due to tight psoas and weak abdominal muscles
Fig. 3   Psoas muscle, a major hip flexor

type of muscular imbalance. Running repeatedly contracts the psoas to lift the legs with each stride and tightens the outer back muscles. The psoas muscle and the muscles connected to the back work much more than the abdominal muscles. So unless you work to strengthen the stomach area, running promotes a basic structural imbalance characterized by a tight psoas and back, and weak abdominals.

Leg Lifts can strengthen the stomach if done correctly. They will strain the back if done incorrectly. Lie in Mountain Pose and elongate your spine. Do not allow your spine to overarch while doing Leg Lifts. Overarching is characterized by the rib cage poking up and the space under the waist increasing while lowering the legs. If your back does overarch, it means that your legs are being lifted by the psoas, a deep abdominal muscle. Activate the abdominals to keep the torso stabilized in an elongated position. Working any other way reinforces an imbalance and may be dangerous.

Don't do the full body sit-ups that used to be taught in school. The rationale for sit-ups is that they strengthen the abdominals. But when doing traditional sit-ups, the muscles that flex the hip do the major part of the work. The abdominal muscles can flex the torso about 30 degrees; to lift higher into a full sit-up, the hip flexors must be contracted. This may strain the psoas muscle, which is designed to lift the thighbone, but not the torso, which is much heavier.

Instead of the classical sit-ups, use the variations given here. As in Leg Lifts (Urdhva Prasarita Padasana), always keep the spine stabilized in an elongated position. When you can do Leg Lifts and Yoga Sit-Ups without strain, and you understand how to protect your back, begin practicing Boat Pose (Navasana).

URDHVA PRASARITA PADASANA

LEG LIFTS

1. Placement. Lie on the back in Mountain Pose, palms down. Relax your neck and throat. If your chin is above your forehead, place a folded towel under your head so your chin is parallel to the floor.

2. Preparation. Bend both knees and place your feet parallel and near your sitting bones. Bend your right knee in toward your chest. Exhale and firm the abdomen to stabilize the pelvis. Extend through the right heel. Exhale and lower your right leg to the floor slowly and with control. Practice on the opposite side. Build to ten repetitions with each leg. Reverse the movement sequence by extending the heel of the bent leg on the floor until the leg is straight, and lift the leg to a vertical position. Then bend the knee in toward the chest, and place the foot on the floor. Build to ten repetitions with each leg.

3. Preparation. Do #2, bending the right leg but keeping the left leg straight and on the floor. Pay attention not to push off with this leg or the back of the head. Build to ten repetitions with each leg.

4. Preparation. When you can do #1, #2, and #3 comfortably, practice with both legs straight. Begin in #1. Exhale, firm the abdominal muscles to maintain the length of the spine, and lift one leg to 90 degrees. Extend through the heel. Exhale as you slowly lower the leg. Increase strength by holding each raised leg at 90, 60, and 30 degrees for a full breath. Then practice lifting and lowering both legs together (Urdhva Prasarita Padasana, described in #6.).

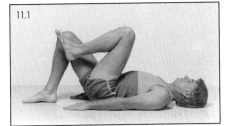
11.1

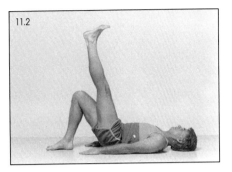
11.2

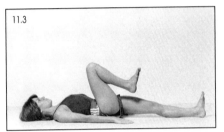
11.3

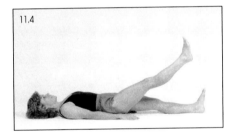
11.4

11.1 Leg Lifts–both knees bent
11.2 Leg Lifts–straighten raised leg
11.3 Leg Lifts–leg on floor straight
11.4 Leg Lifts–both legs straight

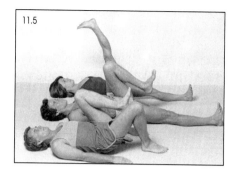

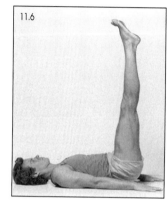

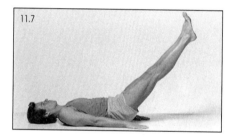

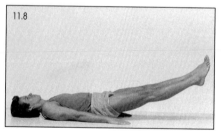

5. Note. Because it may be confusing to see how these three Leg Lifts differ, here is a picture of all three variations. First, both legs bend; second, only one leg bends; finally, both legs are straight throughout.

6. Pose. Lie in Mountain Pose. Exhale and elongate your spine by stretching out through your heels and head. Then without overarching your lower back, lift both legs to 90 degrees. Hold for a full breath. Exhale, lower both legs to 60 degrees, and hold for a full breath. Exhale, lower both legs to 30 degrees, and hold for a full breath. Exhale lower both legs to supine Mountain Pose. As your strength increases, lift your legs to 30 degrees, 60 degrees, and 90 degrees and hold for longer and longer periods. Eventually do the pose with your arms stretched overhead on the floor behind you.

Benefits: All variations of Leg Lifts (Urdhva Prasarita Padasana) strengthen the abdomen and back.

11.5 Leg Lifts–three variations
11.6 Leg Lifts–legs at 90 degrees
11.7 Leg Lifts–legs at 60 degrees
11.8 Leg Lifts–legs at 30 degrees

YOGA SIT-UPS

1. Placement. Lie on your back with your knees bent and your feet placed parallel to each other on a wall. Be far enough from the wall so that your shin-bones and thighbones form a right angle. Cross the arms over the chest, and hold each elbow with the opposite hand.

2. Pose. Exhale and tuck your chin to your chest. Firm your abdominal muscles to lift your head and upper back off the floor, one vertebra at a time. Keep your shoulders drawn away from your ears. Breathe evenly as you lift with control and lower with control. As with stretching, never jerk.

3. Variation. Begin as in #1. Interlace your fingers behind your head. Exhale and, contracting your abdominals, roll your head and upper back up as in #2. Flex your hips, taking your feet off the wall, and touch your elbows to your thighs. Place your toes back on the wall and lower your upper back, but do not place your head on the floor. Firm your abdominals again and repeat the exercise. Begin by doing two or three, working up to ten.

4. Variation. To strengthen the oblique abdominal muscles, begin as in #3, with the feet on the wall. Flex the hips as in #3, but cross the right elbow to touch the left knee, and then cross the left elbow to the right knee. Release by placing your toes back on the wall, and lower your upper back, keeping your head lifted. Repeat as many times as possible without strain, remembering that it's the elbows that cross, not the knees.

Benefits: Yoga Sit-Ups strengthen the neck and stomach, and protect the back. People with swayback posture can benefit from doing these regularly.

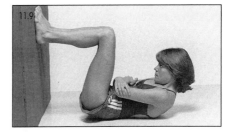

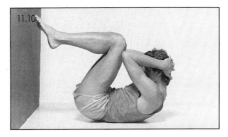

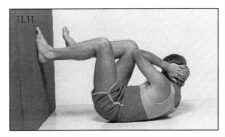

11.9   Yoga Sit-Ups–arms across chest
11.10 Yoga Sit-Ups–elbows to knees
11.11 Yoga Sit-Ups–elbow to opposite knee

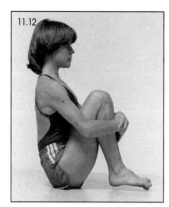

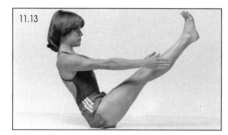

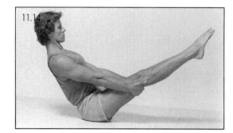

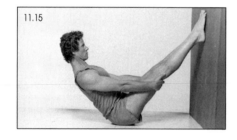

11.12 Boat Pose–placement
11.13 Boat Pose
11.14 Boat Pose–hands supporting
       legs
11.15 Boat Pose–feet against wall

NAVASANA

BOAT POSE

1. Placement. Sit in Staff Pose. Bend your knees in toward your chest. Exhale and lift your feet slightly off the floor, wrapping your arms around your shins. Balance on your sitting bones, back erect.

2. Pose. Exhale and extend through your heels as you straighten both legs, keeping your feet and knees together. Remember to breathe! Extend your arms alongside your body, parallel to the floor and with the palms facing in. Open the chest by drawing the shoulders away from the ears and lifting the sternum (breastbone) toward the head. Balance forward on your sitting bones and not back on your sacrum or lower back. Hold for a few full breaths, bend your knees, and bring your feet down on the floor. Release back into Staff Pose.

3. Variation. Practice #1. Exhale and extend your legs as in #2, supporting just above the backs of your knees with both hands. Use the arms as levers to help open the chest and lengthen the spine. Balance on your sitting bones and not on your sacrum or lower back.

4. Aid. Sit on your mat in Staff Pose, facing a wall. Place your feet on the wall so your heels are level with your eyes. Place the hands behind the knees, and lean back until the torso is at a right angle to the legs. When you can balance, let go of your legs and bring your arms as in #2.

Caution: Do not attempt Boat Pose if you have a weak lower back.

Benefits: Boat Pose (Navasana) strengthens the back, the abdomen, and the legs.

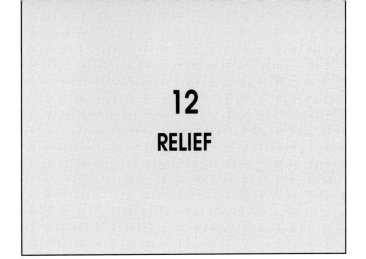

12
RELIEF

BACK STRETCHES

There are two major areas that runners and other athletes should stretch: the legs, which may be self-evident, and the back, an area frequently ignored.

Anatomically there are several salient facts relating to the back and running. Between the bones of the spine there are discs, hydraulic "shock absorbers," that allow for movement and compression. They account for the shape of the back and for one-fourth of its length. Somewhere around a person's twenty-fifth year, the arteries and the veins stop feeding into these discs. They then get their nutrition from the vertebrae and from their ability to absorb nutrients from surrounding tissues. The more movement in the back, the more opportunity there is for the discs to absorb nutrients and to maintain their hydraulic, elastic, and stress-absorbing qualities.

Traversing the front and back of the spine, from top to bottom, are two long ligaments that support the spine. These ligaments keep the discs and the bones aligned by preventing excessive movement. Ligaments, like other connective tissues, contain microorgans that contract but do not expand. If these ligaments are not stretched, they stay contracted. When a person runs he or she is jumping vertically from foot to foot, with overall momentum downward, due to gravity. The effect on

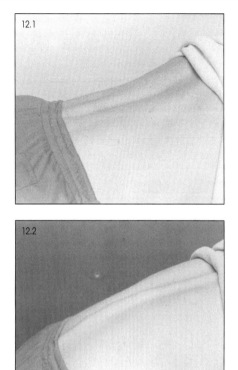

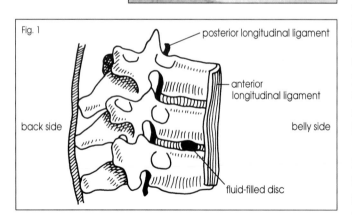

12.1   Back Stretch–correct
       position
12.2   Back Stretch–incorrect
       position: vertebrae
       protruding

Fig. 1   Side view: intervertebral
        discs

the back, and particularly on the spinal discs, is one of compression. So for the health of the back, stretching is essential to lengthen the ligaments, which encase the discs. This lengthening will allow the discs to return to a more plump, fuller state. And stretching creates more space between the vertebrae, thus deterring the flattening of the discs.

Evaluating the Elongation of the Back

To stretch your back safely it must first be positioned correctly, so that the four natural curves of your back are preserved. To understand this, do the following exercise. Place a book on a tabletop and stand about two feet away, with your feet parallel and hips' width apart. Bend forward from your hips and place your hands on the table, straddling the book. Activate your thighs and make the front of your torso long by moving your pubic bone away from your chest. Move the base of the skull and the shoulders away from each other. Now place the fingertips of one hand on the back of your waist. The back is properly elongated when the spine is gently indented. If the vertebrae poke up, move the pubic bone back farther and lift the tailbone and buttocks higher. If your hamstrings are tight, this may not be possible. In this case raise the torso higher until the vertebrae fall into proper alignment: you will feel a channel where the spine lies. To stand, treat the spine as one unit, like a yardstick, and come up by moving the pelvis forward and the chest upright. When you treat your spine as a single unit you avoid placing undue stress on your lower back.

Caution: The first four poses in this chapter lengthen the spine, and are safe for everyone to practice. The next three poses stretch and relax tight back muscles. In the final two poses the spine is compressed, particularly if the back is chronically tense. If you have a herniated disc, practice the first four poses, the fifth pose (Knees-to-Chest Pose) as described in #2, but do not do the Spinal Rolls until your symptoms disappear.

DOORKNOB STRETCH I

1. Placement. Stand in Mountain Pose. Hold onto two knobs of an open door (or the lip of a sink), and step back until your torso is parallel to the floor. Keep the arms straight and the throat and abdomen relaxed, and allow the head to be a natural extension of the spine. Place one hand on your back to see if the vertebrae at the back of your waist poke out. If they do, practice as in #3.

2. Pose. Ask a partner to place his or her hands on your hips and gently draw back. The partner protects his or her own back by keeping his or her back lengthened and bending at the knees. For greater leverage the assistant can place a soft belt, tie, or towel around your hips.

3. Variation. If your hamstrings are simply too tight to bring your back into proper alignment, eliminate the stretch on your hamstrings by kneeling. The assisting person then squats or sits in Diamond Pose (Chapter 8), takes hold of your hips with his or her hands or a belt, and leans back.

Benefits: Doorknob Stretch I stretches the back and hamstrings, and opens the chest and shoulders.

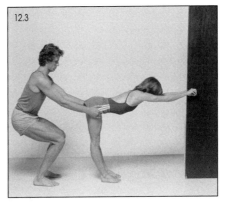

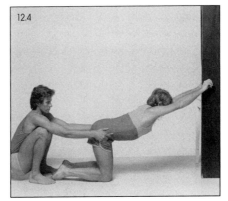

12.3   Doorknob Stretch I–standing
12.4   Doorknob Stretch I–kneeling

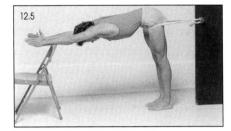

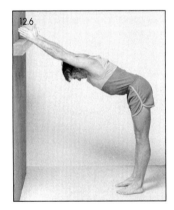

12.5   Doorknob Stretch II
12.6   Doorknob Stretch II–using a
        ledge

DOORKNOB STRETCH II

1. Placement. For this version of Doorknob Stretch you need a cloth belt or tie, a chair, and a door. Tie the ends of the belt or tie together, and wrap it around the knobs of an open door. Place the chair in front of you. Step inside the belt and stand with your back to the door. Place the belt at the front hip crease and stand so the belt is taut. Stand with your feet parallel and hips' width apart, and lift your kneecaps.

2. Pose. Inhale and stretch your arms overhead. Exhale and bend from the hip crease, placing your forearms on the back of the chair. With one hand touch the back of your waist to make sure your vertebrae are not poking out. If bones poke up, bend your knees and lift your sitting bones, or place your hands on a higher prop as in #3. Lengthen from your tailbone through your fingertips. Hold for twenty to thirty seconds, breathing evenly. Gradually build time in the pose to one to two minutes. As your hamstrings stretch, place your arms on the seat or lower rungs of the chair.

3. Variation. Face a ledge (maybe the top of a refrigerator or the door of a bathroom stall), standing an arm's length away. Place your wrists on the ledge, and then walk your feet back until you are bent at the hips and your legs are directly under your hips. Place your feet parallel to each other and activate your legs. On an exhalation extend your fingers outward, move your pubic bone away from your chest, and lift your sitting bones. Pause on an inhalation and on an exhalation deepen the stretch. Do for five or six breaths. To release, walk toward the ledge as you stand, and then lower your arms.

Benefits: Doorknob Stretch II lengthens the spine, rejuvenates discs, and stretches the chest and shoulders. It is also an excellent way to learn correct forward bending.

FULL BODY STRETCH

1. Placement. Lie on your back in Mountain Pose. If your chin is higher than your forehead, place a folded towel under your head. Inhale and stretch your arms overhead on the floor. Draw your shoulders away from your ears.

2. Pose. Keep your face, neck, and throat relaxed as you stretch from your heels through your fingertips. Pause on an inhalation; stretch on an exhalation. Repeat the pose for five or six breaths. To release, bring your arms to your sides, bend your knees, and place your feet on the floor.

3. Variation. Stretch one side at a time. Exhale and stretch the right heel and right hand away from each other. Inhale and pause. Exhale and stretch the left heel and left hand away from each other. Repeat three or four times to each side.

Benefits: Full Body Stretch stretches the entire body and aligns the spine. Use this pose between supine poses to realign the body. It is also excellent to practice before or after Corpse Pose (Chapter 20).

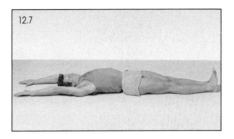

12.7   Full Body Stretch

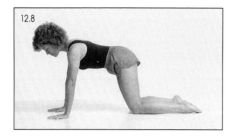

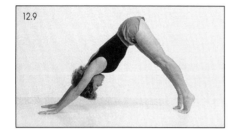

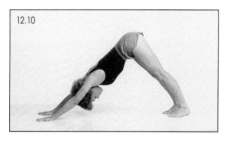

12.8 Downward-Facing Dog
      Pose–placement
12.9 Downward-Facing Dog
      Pose–preparation on toes
12.10 Downward-Facing Dog
      Pose

ADHO MUKHA SVANASANA

DOWNWARD-FACING DOG POSE

1. Placement. Kneel on all fours. Place your hands and knees directly opposite each other, with your hands shoulders' width apart and your knees directly under your hips. Turn your toes under. To avoid an uneven stretch in the feet, don't allow the heels to drop out, but keep the heels above your toes. Relax your throat and abdomen and draw your shoulders away from your ears.

2. Pose. Exhale and lift your sitting bones toward the ceiling as you straighten your legs. Stay high up on the toes. Press the hands into the floor, lengthening through the index fingers, as you continue to move the sitting bones away from the breastbone. Keep your kneecaps lifted. Continue to relax your throat and abdomen. Maintaining this alignment, lower your heels toward the floor. Hold for ten to fifteen seconds, breathing evenly. Slowly increase your length of time in the pose to two minutes. To release, come back to kneeling on all fours. Gently sit back on your heels and, with your arms stretched out in front of you, lower your torso and forehead to the floor. (You may want to put a towel under your forehead.) Rest for several breaths. Come to a sitting position.

3. Aid. Kneel an arm's length away from a chair that is against a wall. Place your hands on the chair seat and turn your toes under. Press your hands into the chair seat as you lift your sitting bones to straighten your legs. Stay up on your toes as in #2. Lengthen your spine, relax your throat, and broaden your abdomen. Maintaining length in the spine, slowly lower the heels to the floor. Hold for fifteen seconds, breathing evenly. Gradually increase your time in the pose. To release, come back to a kneeling position and fold your arms, placing them on the chair seat. Sit back on your heels and rest your forehead on your arms for several breaths. When ready, come to a sitting position.

4. Aid. Kneel on all fours, bracing your hands against a wall or step. Follow directions for #1 and #2, pressing equally on the inside and outside of each hand.

Benefits: Downward-Facing Dog Pose (Adho Mukha Svanasana) is a perfect pose for runners, both before and after running. It stretches the entire back side of the body, especially the hamstrings, calves, and Achilles tendons. It also strengthens the upper body, opens the chest, and improves breathing.

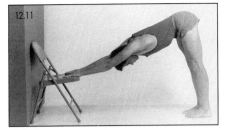

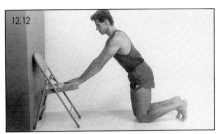

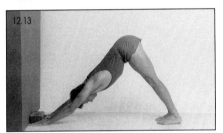

12.11 Downward-Facing Dog
      Pose–placement with chair
12.12 Downward-Facing Dog
      Pose–hands on chair
12.13 Downward-Facing Dog
      Pose–with block at wall

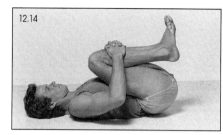

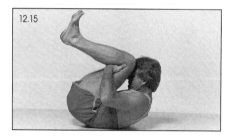

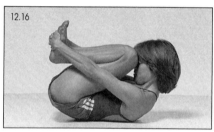

12.14 Knees-to-Chest Pose–with hands on shins
12.15 Knees-to-Chest Pose–with hands behind thighs
12.16 Knees-to-Chest Pose–with hands around feet

KNEES-TO-CHEST POSE

1. Placement. Lie on your back in Mountain Pose. If your chin is higher than your forehead, place a folded towel under your head. Bend your knees and place your heels close to your sitting bones. Exhale and bend the knees in toward the chest, interlacing the fingers below the knees.

2. Pose. Exhale and extend through the heels. Release your abdomen and relax your throat as your draw your knees closer to your chest. Hold for ten to twenty seconds, breathing evenly. To release, lower your feet back to the floor and slowly straighten your legs back to Mountain Pose.

3. Variation. To decrease the stretch, or if your knees are injured, place your hands on your thighs under your folded knees. Draw your legs in, and on an exhalation, lift your forehead to your knees. Hold five to ten seconds and release. This is excellent to do after Shoulderstand (Chapter 16). It releases tension in the lower back and neck.

4. Variation. Increase the stretch by interlacing your fingers behind the balls of your feet. Lift the head to the knees on an exhalation. Inhale as you release.

Caution: People with a herniated disc should not attempt #3 and #4. Instead do the pose as described in #2, gently squeezing the knees into the chest while stretching the pubic bone down away from the sternum.

Benefits: Knees-to-Chest Pose (Apanasana) stretches the entire back, particularly the lower back.

SPINAL ROLL

1. Placement. Sit on a well-padded mat. Bend your knees and place your feet on the floor. Interlace your fingers behind your knees. Place the forehead on or near the knees.

2. Pose. Keep your body in this position, and on an exhalation, slowly lean back. Gently rock back and forth betweeen your buttocks and your shoulders. Allow the legs to create a free-swinging momentum.

3. Variation. After rolling back and forth ten or more times, rest on your shoulders and upper back, breathing evenly. In this holding position the knees will be on the forehead. Exhale and roll up to sitting.

4. Variation. After your back has gained some flexibility, hold in #3. On an exhalation straighten one leg at a time and hold for 10 seconds, breathing evenly. Then on an exhalation straighten both legs so the tips of the toes are on the floor behind you. Hold for ten seconds, breathing evenly. Bend your knees back to your forehead and slowly roll down.

Caution: This pose is contraindicated for people with a herniated disc.

Benefits: Spinal Roll is a gentle warm-up for the back and legs. It also relieves tension in the back.

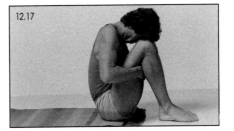

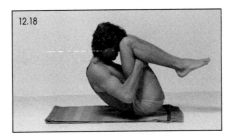

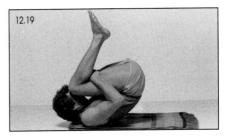

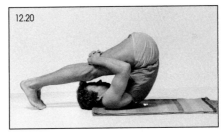

12.17   Spinal Roll–placement
12.18   Spinal Roll–roll onto back
12.19   Spinal Roll–rest on shoulders
12.20   Spinal Roll–straighten legs

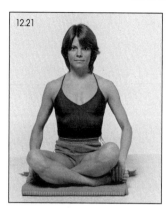

CROSSED-LEG SPINAL ROLL

1. Placement. Sit on a well-padded mat, with the legs crossed at the ankles. Hold the top of your left foot with your right hand; hold the top of your right foot with your left hand. (The legs are crossed, but the arms are not.)

2. Pose. Inhale and sit tall. Exhale, round the back, and place your forehead to the floor, or as near to it as possible. Maintain this ball position with the body, and inhale as you roll backward on the spine until you are high up on the shoulders. Exhale and roll back to sitting. Then repeat: inhale and sit tall, exhale and place the forehead to floor, and so on.

3. Variation. Do #2 six to ten times. When the back is warmed up, practice as in #2, but straighten the legs as much as possible and place the toes on the floor when you have rolled onto the shoulders. Bend the knees and take hold of the ankles as in #1 to roll up. Practice this entire series again by crossing your legs so the opposite leg is on the bottom when sitting.

Caution: This pose is contraindicated for people with a herniated disc.

Benefits: Crossed-Leg Spinal Roll develops coordination and balance, and warms up and stretches the back.

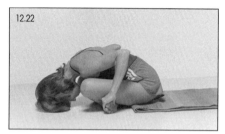

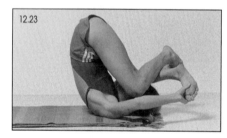

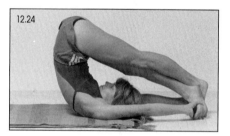

12.21   Crossed-Leg Spinal
         Roll–placement
12.22   Crossed-Leg Spinal
         Roll–head to floor
12.23   Crossed-Leg Spinal Roll–roll
         to shoulders
12.24   Crossed-Leg Spinal
         Roll–straighten legs

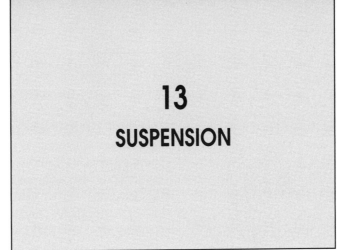

13
SUSPENSION

STANDING FORWARD BENDS

Toe touching is one of the most common ways people stretch. Unfortunately this stretch is usually executed incorrectly. Most people don't bend from the hips when attempting to touch their toes, but instead fold forward at the waist, thereby compressing the spine; if done consistently this can be dangerous.

The main reason for doing standing forward bends is to stretch the backs of the legs, the hamstring muscles. These muscles begin at the sitting bones, run down the backs of the thighs, over the backs of the knees, and connect to the lower leg bones. The only way to stretch the hamstrings fully in standing forward bends is to move the sitting bones away from the knees. To do this, stand with straight legs and bend from the hips as though the torso were suspended from the sitting bones. Again, the way most people try to touch their toes is to round the upper back and bend from the waist. Feel the difference for yourself: stand in Mountain Pose and then try it both ways.

Many of our daily activities contribute to the hunched shoulders and rounded upper back posture: reading the newspaper, writing a letter, bicycling, and so on. Continual stretching with a rounded back reinforces this tendency. Two long ligaments support the spine from top to bottom. One ligament supports the

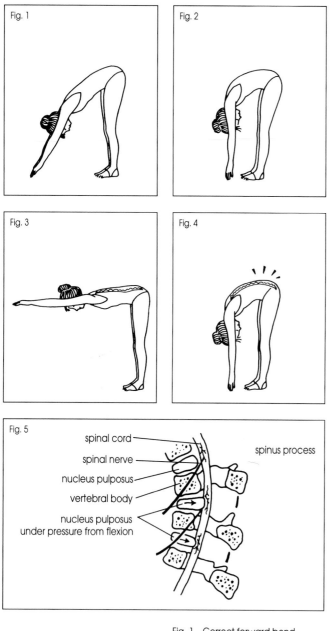

Fig. 1
Fig. 2
Fig. 3
Fig. 4
Fig. 5

spinal cord
spinal nerve
nucleus pulposus
vertebral body
nucleus pulposus
under pressure from flexion
spinus process

Fig. 1   Correct forward bend
Fig. 2   Incorrect forward bend
Fig. 3   Spine fully extended
Fig. 4   Lower back stressed
Fig. 5   Pressure on discs results
          from improper forward
          bending

posterior, or back side, of the spine, and the other ligament supports the anterior, or belly side, of the spine. If you round your back to touch your toes, the posterior ligament stretches, but the anterior one contracts. Unless this imbalance is counteracted, the ligaments of the back become uneven in length, causing the back to curve forward even more and the strength of the back to dissipate.

Furthermore, the hamstring muscles are usually stronger than the back. If you start tugging on the two simultaneously, injury is more likely to occur in the back. Incorrect forward bending places tremendous pressure on the spinal discs, because the front edges of the vertebrae are squeezed together, forcing the nuclei of the discs backward into the spinal cord.

All of this can be avoided by learning to bend forward correctly. Here is the most important principle: when bending forward, whether you are standing or sitting, consider the torso a single unit and bend from the hips. To do this, stretch the pubic bone away from the chest, with the buttocks stretching away from the knees. This strengthens and protects the back. When tilting the pelvis forward, the front of the torso must be lengthened to prevent the back from rounding. When the back is one unit, no one curve of the spine is reversing against its natural shape, so the discs and vertebrae are not forced out of alignment.

Before beginning these poses, read the instructions at the beginning of Chapter 12 for evaluating the elongation of the back. Apply this test to all standing forward bends at the horizontal position. This will ensure that the spine is lengthened. When bending forward to place the stomach on the thighs, the bones of the back will probably poke out. It is important that the bones poke out gently and uniformly. If one or more bones protrude in an obvious way, lift the torso until greater uniformity is achieved.

UTTANASANA, VARIATION

WALL HANG

1. Placement. Stand in Mountain Pose, with your back against a wall. Place the feet about eight inches from the wall and hips' width apart. Lift your kneecaps up. Place your hands on your front groins. It is from the front groins that you will bend forward.

2. Preparation. Exhale and treat the entire spine as one unit as you begin to bend the torso forward. Allow your buttocks to move up the wall. Lengthen the front of your torso. Touch the spine at the back of the waist. If the vertebrae poke up above the muscles, then lift the entire torso higher in order to maintain the natural curves of the spine.

3. Pose. Now allow the back to round down very gently, aiming the top of the head to the floor, not to the knees. Let your arms and head hang. If your hands touch the floor, hold each elbow with the opposite hand. Feel gravity draw you down. Relax your abdomen and allow the muscles and ligaments of your back to lengthen. Hold for fifteen seconds, breathing evenly. Gradually increase your time in the pose to one minute. To come up, place your hands on your thighs and bring your torso back to #2. Then, moving your spine as a unit, lift your torso to the wall.

4. Variation. Practice #3, holding each elbow with the opposite hand. Lift the elbows out toward the center of the room. With each breath, stretch the armpits toward the floor. This will help you to lengthen the spine. To come up, release your arms and lift your torso to the wall.

Benefits: Wall Hang (Uttanasana, variation) is a marvelous way to learn proper forward bending, because you can feel the buttocks move up the wall. The backs of the legs are given a wonderful stretch.

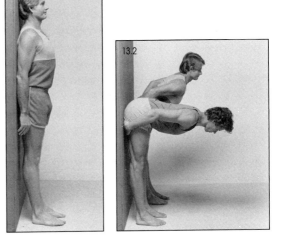

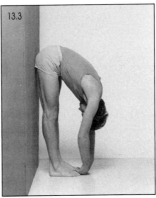

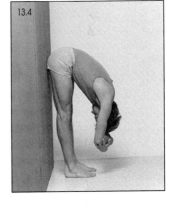

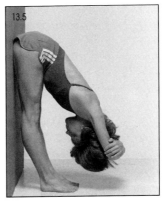

13.1   Wall Hang–placement
13.2   Wall Hang–preliminary
        movement
13.3   Wall Hang
13.4   Wall Hang–holding elbows
13.5   Wall Hang–lifted elbows

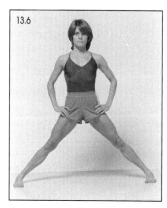

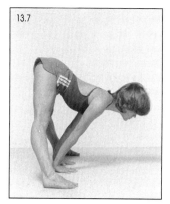

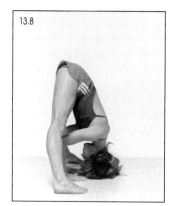

PRASARITA PADOTTANASANA

SPREAD-FOOT FORWARD BEND

1. Placement. Stand in Mountain Pose. Exhale and with a jump separate your feet approximately five feet apart. Keep your feet parallel and your thighs active. Place the hands at the front groins.

2. Pose. Exhale and, moving the torso as one unit, bend forward from the hip creases. Exhale and place your hands on the floor, shoulders' width apart and in line with your feet. Inhale and lift the head as you also lift the buttocks to lengthen the back. Relax your abdomen. Exhale, bend the elbows back between the knees and place the top of your head on the floor. In this position your lower arm bones will be at right angles to your upper arm bones. Hold for ten to twenty seconds, breathing evenly. To release, reverse the procedure: straighten your arms first and then lift your torso as a unit. Jump your feet back to Mountain Pose.

13.6   Spread-Foot Forward
        Bend–placement
13.7   Spread-Foot Forward
        Bend–hands on floor
13.8   Spread-Foot Forward Bend

3. Variation. Bring your hands behind your back and interlace your fingers. Keep the front spine elongated and the chest broad. Exhale, bend at the hips, and bring the torso as far forward as possible, keeping the spine lengthened. Lift your arms away from your buttocks. Exhale, allow your back to round gently, and extend the top of your head toward the floor, bringing your arms as far overhead as possible. Hold for fifteen to twenty seconds, breathing evenly. Inhale and come to standing. If you can't interlace your fingers behind you, hold a pole or cloth. Faithful practice will enable you to bring your hands together.

4. Aid. Place a chair two to two and one-half feet in front of you. Follow the same directions as in #2, except place your hands on the seat of the chair rather than the floor. If you cannot fully lengthen the spine, place the hands on the back of the chair. To release, bend your knees, and, placing your hands on your thighs, lift your torso so it is parallel to the floor. Elongate the spine and then stand erect by lifting the torso as a unit.

Benefits: Spread-Foot Forward Bend (Prasarita Padottanasana) stretches the hamstrings and inner thighs. It also strengthens the legs and ankles, and is excellent for relieving upper body tension.

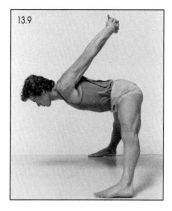

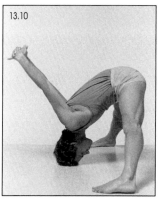

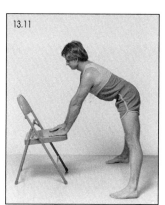

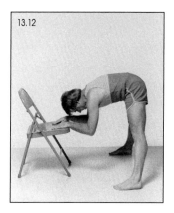

13.9   Spread-Foot Forward
       Bend–arms extended back
13.10 Spread-Foot Forward
       Bend–head to floor
13.11 Spread-Foot Forward Bend
       with hands on chair–
       placement
13.12 Spread-Foot Forward Bend
       with hands on chair

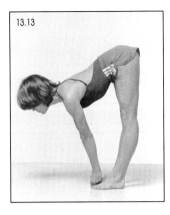

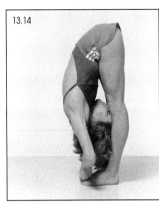

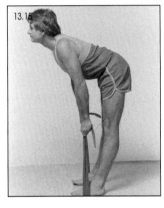

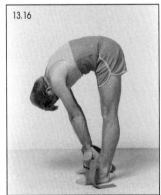

13.13 Standing Toe-Holding
Pose–head lifted and back
extended
13.14 Standing Toe-Holding
Pose–head to shins
13.15 Standing Toe-Holding
Pose–back extended using
belt
13.16 Standing Toe-Holding
Pose–forward bend using
belt

PADANGUSTHASANA

STANDING TOE-HOLDING POSE

1. Placement. Stand in Mountain Pose and separate your feet approximately one foot apart. Lift your kneecaps and keep your thighs active.

2. Pose. Exhale, bend forward from the hip creases, and grasp the big toes with the first two fingers and the thumbs so that the palms face each other. Straighten the arms, lift the head, and lift the buttocks high. Move your shoulders away from your ears. Relax your abdomen. Exhale, bend the elbows out to the sides, and lengthen the spine toward the floor so the head comes to the shins. Hold for ten seconds, breathing evenly. Release by straightening the arms, and come back to standing on an inhalation. Return to Mountain Pose.

3. Aid. Place a belt or strap under the arches of the feet. Exhale, bend forward, and grasp the belt with both hands. Straighten your legs and arms. Stretch your buttocks upward. Look up and lift the torso high enough to draw the vertebrae at the back of the waist in. Keep lengthening the spine. Exhale, bend the elbows out to the sides, and lengthen the top of the head toward the floor. Hold for two full breaths. Drop the belt, bend the knees, place the hands on the thighs, and elongate the spine by lifting the torso and moving the pubic bone away from the chest. Once the spine is elongated, come to a standing position with the knees still bent by lifting the spine as a unit.

Benefits: Standing Toe-Holding Pose (Padangusthasana) stretches the legs and lengthens the spine.

UTTANASANA

STANDING FORWARD BEND

1. Placement. Stand in Mountain Pose.

2. Pose. Inhale and lift your arms overhead, with your palms facing forward. Lower the shoulders away from the ears throughout. Exhale, bend forward from the hip creases, and place the hands on the floor beside the feet. Lift your buttocks. If your weight is heavy on your heels, move your weight forward onto the balls of your feet, and then redistribute your weight over your feet. Exhale and lower your head to your shins. Relax your abdomen and keep your throat soft. Hold for two full breaths. Slowly increase your time in the pose to one minute. To come up, first lift the head, and then lift your torso as a unit.

3. Variation. To increase the stretch, begin in #2 and move your hands farther back and behind your feet, with your fingertips in a line and pointing forward. Ideally your hips are directly over your feet. Lift the buttocks high and open the backs of the legs. Keep your arms straight and active. Relax your throat and abdomen. As you gain flexibility, practice with your palms resting on the floor.

4. Variation. To intensify the stretch, place the right forearm on the right calf and the left forearm on the left calf. Relax your throat and abdomen. Move your shoulders away from your ears. Exhale and draw the torso toward the legs. Hold for five seconds, breathing evenly. Gradually increase your time in the pose to thirty seconds.

5. Aid. If your hands don't touch the floor, place books by the sides of your feet as shown. Bend forward and place your hands on the books, fingers pointing forward, and proceed as in #2. Be sure to keep your legs active and buttocks lifted.

Benefits: Standing Forward Bend (Uttanasana) stretches the entire back side of the body.

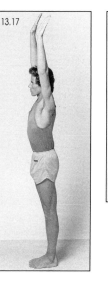
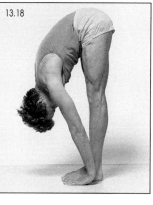

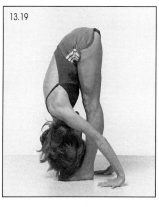
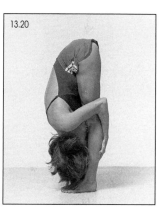

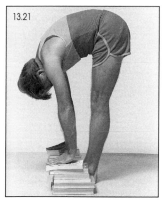

13.17 Standing Forward Bend–placement with arms overhead

13.18 Standing Forward Bend–hands beside feet

13.19 Standing Forward Bend–hands behind feet

13.20 Standing Forward Bend–forearms on calves

13.21 Standing Forward Bend–hands on books

14
DON'T BE GIRDLED

POSES FOR THE UPPER BACK, SHOULDERS, AND ARMS

Runners sometimes concentrate so much on the lower body that the chest, shoulders, and arms remain underdeveloped. A weak upper body taxes the lower body by making it work harder to carry and balance a dull torso. Such imbalanced development can lead to a stiff shoulder girdle, with a tense neck, a concave chest, and weak arms.

Focusing on the upper back, shoulders, and arms in your yoga practice can, therefore, be very helpful. This chapter includes exercises and postures to benefit the upper back, shoulders, and arms. A special caution about the push-up poses described in this chapter: these exercises develop the arms and strengthen the abdomen, but some athletes should do only a moderate number of push-ups, focusing more on stretching the abdomen. An overly tight abdomen acts as a lever on the chest, pulling the rib cage down. The chest becomes flat and lifeless, and the lung capacity is limited. Usually the head will protrude also. When the chest is collapsed, the back muscles lose tone because they are always extended. The whole body loses balance. Look in the mirror. If you tend toward this pattern, alter your exercises to make yourself truly balanced and fit, not just hard. Do fewer push-ups, leg lifts, and sit-ups, and do more backbending poses.

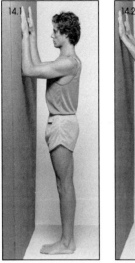

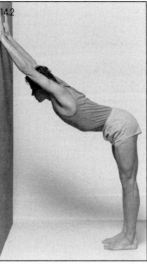

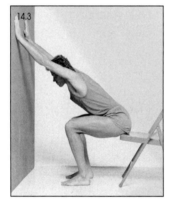

14.1   Chest Opener–placement
14.2   Chest Opener
14.3   Chest Opener–seated in
         chair

As you do the following exercises, observe your face, throat, and arms, and allow these areas to remain soft and relaxed. As the upper back, shoulders, and arms become stronger and more flexible, the chest can open. Deeper, freer breathing will result. Liberating your breath means longer, stronger runs and the ability to do more challenging workouts.

CHEST OPENER

1. Placement. Stand in Mountain Pose, facing a wall, with your feet parallel and hips' width apart. Place your hands on the wall, shoulders' width apart, with your middle fingers vertical. (If your shoulders are stiff, your hands may turn out. As your flexibility increases, you will be able to place your hands vertically.) Walk back until your arms are fully extended and your legs are perpendicular to the floor.

2. Pose. Exhale. Keeping your arms straight and without moving your hands, turn your inner elbows up. Lift your sitting bones up and lengthen the front of your torso. Your legs remain perpendicular to your torso throughout. Keep the kneecaps lifted and the arms extended. Hold for several even breaths. To release, take a step toward the wall and return to Mountain Pose.

3. Aid. If tight hamstrings prevent you from doing #2 with straight legs, sit in a chair facing a wall and practice as in #2.

Benefits: Chest Opener opens the shoulders and stretches the legs. It also strengthens the arms, upper back, and chest.

HANDCLASP SHOULDER STRETCH

1. Placement. Stand in Mountain Pose. Interlace your fingers behind your back.

2. Pose. Move both hands to the left, placing the back of your right hand against your left rib cage. Exhale, lower the shoulders, and draw the shoulder blades together and down. The left elbow moves in toward the spine and down. Breathe high into the chest and lift the spine with each inhalation. Hold for fifteen to twenty seconds, breathing evenly. Practice to the opposite side and return to Mountain Pose.

Benefits: Handclasp Shoulder Stretch stretches the chest, strengthens the upper back, and adds mobility to the shoulder girdle.

PARVATASANA

ARM STRETCH

1. Placement. Sit on your heels (Diamond Pose, Chapter 8). If this is difficult, sit on one or more firmly folded blankets, or stand with your feet parallel and hips' width apart. Interlock the fingers, with the right thumb on top.

2. Pose. Exhale, maintaining the interlock, and extend the arms overhead, turning the palms to face the ceiling. Soften your face and throat as you continue lifting evenly on both sides of the body. Hold for ten seconds, breathing evenly. Release your arms and change the interlock of your fingers so your left thumb is on top. Repeat.

3. Variation. If you are standing, note that although the feet are apart, the body remains in Mountain Pose. Stretch the arms and keep the face and throat soft.

4. Aid. In position #3, hold a tie between your hands. Exhale and stretch your arms overhead, reaching your fists toward the ceiling. Stretch the inner elbows and keep the tension on the tie. If your shoulders are tight, your arms may not be vertical. As you gain flexibility, move your hands in toward the center.

Benefits: Arm Stretch (Parvatasana) strengthens the upper arms and stretches the shoulders.

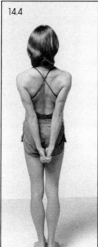
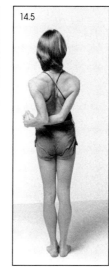

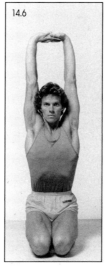
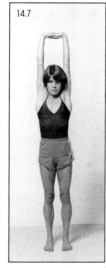
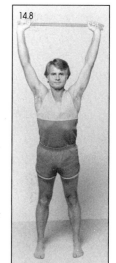

14.4 Handclasp Shoulder
Stretch–placement
14.5 Handclasp Shoulder Stretch
14.6 Arm Stretch
14.7 Arm Stretch–standing
14.8 Arm Stretch–with tie

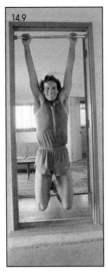

BAR HANG

1. Placement. Wrap your hands around a secure exercise bar placed at the upper edge of a doorway.

2. Pose. Exhale, relax your knees, and, with your arms straight, let your body weight hang from your hands. Breathe evenly and let the back stretch out. As you get more experienced you can bend your knees enough to take your feet off the floor.

3. Variation. Hold the bar but turn your hands so your palms face back. Broaden the space between your shoulder blades as you hang from your hands. Breathe evenly and let the weight of the body stretch the shoulders and back.

Benefits: Hanging from a bar is a great stretch for the back, shoulders, and arms. It is an especially good pose for baseball players, tennis players, and all other athletes who continually tighten the upper body.

WRIST STRETCH

1. Placement. Stand in Mountain Pose, facing a wall. Bend your arms and place your palms on the wall, with your fingers pointing toward the floor. Don't be discouraged if this is difficult at first. The tighter the wrists, the farther down the wall the hands are placed.

2. Pose. On each exhalation lean gently into the hands, trying to flatten the entire palms on the wall. As your flexibility increases, move your hands higher up the wall.

Benefits: Wrist Stretch increases flexibility in the wrists.

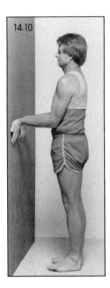
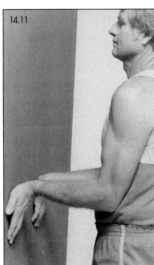

14.9   Bar Hang
14.10 Wrist Stretch–placement
14.11 Wrist Stretch

GOMUKHASANA
COW'S FACE POSE

1. Placement. Sit in Hero Pose (Chapter 8). Distribute the weight evenly on both buttocks.

2. Pose. Stretch both arms down, with your palms turned out and your shoulders blades moving down your back. Exhale, bend your left arm, and place your left hand on your back, palm facing out. Keep the left shoulder down and back and stretch the fingers up. Exhale and extend your right arm overhead. Maintain the stretch of the right arm as you bend it and grasp the left hand with the right. Keep the spine lengthening, shoulders level, and collarbones broad. Relax your throat and soften your gaze. Hold for ten to fifteen seconds, breathing evenly. Release your hands down to your sides, and practice to the opposite side.

3. Variation. Do the pose sitting on your heels (Diamond Pose, Chapter 8). If your knees are tight or your spine collapses, you can place a cushion between your heels and buttocks. Do not be concerned with grasping the hands. The important point is to minimize the disturbance of your legs and torso. Pay attention to your feet, hips, shoulders, throat, and face as you bend your arms. If you experience pain in your knees, practice as in #4.

4. Aid. You can practice this pose standing. Hold a towel, rope, or belt in the right hand and reach for it with the left. Use the towel as a link between your two hands.

Benefits: Cow's Face Pose (Gomukhasana) is excellent for those with rounded shoulders, collapsed chests, or tight arms.

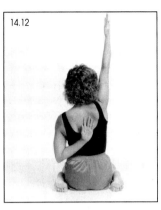

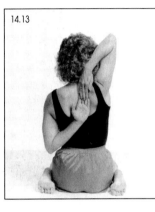

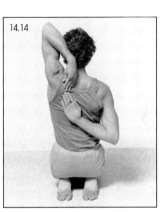

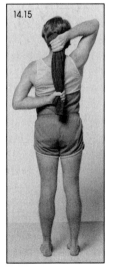

14.12 Cow's Face Pose–placement
14.13 Cow's Face Pose
14.14 Cow's Face Pose–sitting on heels
14.15 Cow's Face Pose–with towel

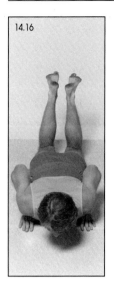

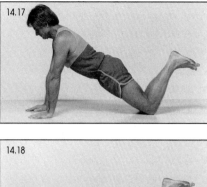

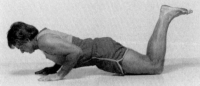

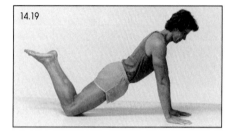

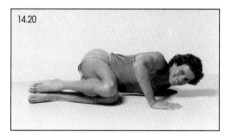

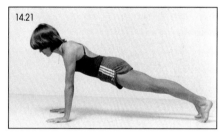

14.16 Yoga Push-Ups–placement with bent knees
14.17 Yoga Push-Ups–lift torso
14.18 Yoga Push-Ups–lower torso
14.19 Yoga Push-Ups–variation for weak arms
14.20 Yoga Push-Ups–getting up
14.21 Yoga Push-Ups–with legs extended

CHATURANGA DANDASANA
YOGA PUSH-UPS

1. Placement. Lie face down on the floor, with your feet one foot apart. Place your hands on the floor and under your shoulders, fingers spread and middle fingers parallel. Keep the elbows close to the body and arms parallel to each other throughout. Bend your knees and bring your heels toward your buttocks.

2. Pose. Lift your torso off the floor. Keep the spine lengthening. Inhale, press evenly on the insides and outsides of the palms, and straighten the arms. Exhale, bend the elbows, and lower the body. Touch only your chest to the floor and repeat. Do as many as you can with the breath even and the face and throat soft. Over time build to ten.

3. Variation. If you can't do one Yoga Push-up, develop your strength by practicing Yoga Push-downs. Begin on your hands and knees. Bring the heels to the buttocks. Exhale, bend your elbows, and lower your body. Roll to one side, pull the knees to the chest, come back to all fours, and begin again.

4. Variation. When you have sufficient strength, straighten your legs, curl your toes under and do full-body push-ups, lifting the lower part of your body as well as the upper. By keeping the elbows close to the body and the palms flat, you will build balanced strength in the arms. Elongate the spine by stretching out through the heels and the crown of the head. Keep the thighs very active.

Benefits: Yoga Push-Ups (Chaturanga Dandasana) (and also Yoga Push-Downs) build strength in the arms and abdomen, and increase mobility in the wrists.

CHATURANGA DANDASANA, VARIATION

CHAIR PUSH-UPS

1. Placement. Place the back of a chair against a wall. Kneel an arm's length away, knees hips' width apart, and place the heels of your hands on the chair seat. Bend your arms and lower your chest to the chair. Straighten your legs so you are on your toes and hands.

2. Pose. With the elbows drawn in next to the body, exhale and straighten the arms. Keep the shoulders away from the ears and keep the chest open. Also, keep the head in line with the body; people tend to reach forward with the head, which misaligns the spine. Inhale and touch your chest, not your nose, to the chair. Repeat as many times as you can, maintaining alignment and keeping the breath even.

Benefits: Chair Push-Ups (Chaturanga Dandasana, variation) strengthen the arms, wrists, shoulders, and abdomen.

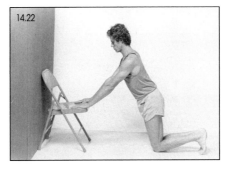

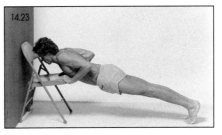

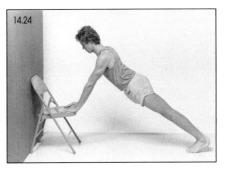

14.22 Chair Push-Ups–placement
14.23 Chair Push-Ups–placement with legs straight
14.24 Chair Push-Ups

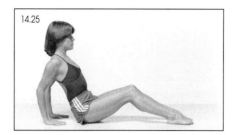

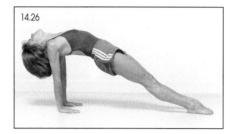

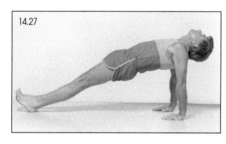

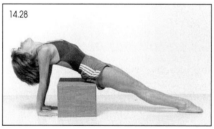

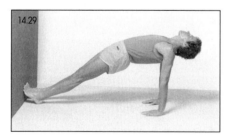

PURVOTTANASANA

INTENSE FRONT STRETCH POSE

1. Placement. Begin in Staff Pose (Chapter 17). Bend your knees enough to place your feet flat on the floor, slightly apart. Eventually, when your knees no longer turn out, you will keep your feet together. Keep your feet parallel and your knees directly in line with your feet, not dropped out to the sides.

2. Pose. Exhale, straighten your arms and legs, and lift your pelvis toward the ceiling. Lengthen the backs of the legs from the buttocks to the heels. Press the soles of the feet to the floor, but do not allow the toes to turn in. Open your chest and, gently drawing your throat in, stretch the base of your skull away from your shoulders. Then drop your head back. Keep the throat soft. Hold for a few full breaths, and gradually increase your time in the pose. Release back to Staff Pose.

3. Variation. Do #2, but instead of balancing on the soles of the feet, work on the heels for a few seconds. Then exhale and stretch the soles of your feet to the floor.

4. Aid. If your arms and shoulders are too weak to support the weight of your body, use a cushion or bench under your buttocks to support some of the weight.

5. Aid. Occasionally work with the toes pushing against a wall to help keep the legs straight. Press solidly on the joints under the big toes to stretch the inner ankles.

Caution: Do not do this pose if you have a neck problem. If your neck is weak, you may compress your cervical spine by taking your head back. To strengthen the neck, learn to lengthen the cervical spine in the standing poses, especially Triangle Pose (Trikonasana).

Benefits: Intense Front Stretch Pose (Purvottanasana) stretches the feet, ankles, and chest. It also strengthens the feet, legs, shoulders, and arms.

14.25 Intense Front Stretch Pose–placement
14.26 Intense Front Stretch Pose
14.27 Intense Front Stretch Pose–on heels
14.28 Intense Front Stretch Pose–buttocks supported
14.29 Intense Front Stretch Pose–toes against wall

15
REJUVENATE

BACKBENDING

Backbending! Even if you're not aware of it, your back yearns to stretch up, out, and over backward. These stretches don't have to be the full-blown backbends of gymnasts; even the simplest backward-bending stretch relieves discomfort, and aligns and strengthens the spine. The reason backbending is good for the spine is that almost all of us, in sitting in our cars or at our desks or before the TV, collapse forward at the waist and thereby push the vertebrae of the spine backward. When the front of the spine collapses, we exert pressure on the discs to move back and into the spinal cord. When the spine collapses, we shorten the muscles at the front of the spine and strain the muscles at the back of the spine, thereby encouraging more collapse. This is a vicious cycle that can lead to back troubles of all kinds.

We need to do the exercises, movements, and stretches that will elongate the back and strengthen back muscles to position the vertebrae one above the other in a long S curve. Each of us can assume a stance where the spine is momentarily elongated, but we can maintain this stance only as long as we think of it. Practicing correct yoga poses builds the natural strength to maintain the correct position of the spine.

Here are some basic guides to practicing healthy backbends:

1. Before and during backbending poses, elongate the spine. Find the spot on your body that is two inches below your navel. Below this spot, gently stretch the pubic bone down. Above this spot lengthen your spine up and press out through the crown of the head. Remember, it is the spine that is lengthening. Do not lift only the front of your chest up, because doing so compresses the back. (For every action there is an opposite and equal reaction.) As the front of the spine elongates it will curve back, and so the chest will naturally open.

2. The legs must be active, that is, the front and particularly the back thigh muscles must contract. The outer thighs lengthen toward the knees. The inner thighs move toward the torso.

3. Keep the front body soft. This includes the front of your groins, your abdomen, and the front of your neck. Visualize softening the entire front of the body right into the front of the spine.

4. Do not be in a hurry to arch your neck back. For several months practice by simply pressing out through the crown of the head. Gently draw the throat into the neck and lengthen the base of the skull away from the shoulders. In this way the front of the neck lends support to the lifting action of the spine. This must be practiced conscientiously before letting the head drop back.

5. As in all yoga, practice so the pose feels right. Always, with or without a teacher, you are responsible for taking care of yourself.

6. After backbending, gently stretch out the hamstrings and the muscles of the lower back by doing Knees-to-Chest (Chapter 12) or Child's Pose (Chapter 20) or both. Gentle twists such as the Crocodile Twist (Chapter 18) and the Simple Twist (Chapter 18) also help to soothe the back after extensive backbending.

Caution: If your back muscles tend to spasm when you do backbending, it means that these muscles are under a lot of stress. Go back to Pelvic Tilting (Chapter 6), back stretches, gentle twisting, and the standing poses. Eventually you will be able to return to backbending; it's just that right now you need more preparation. Just enjoy the feelings of a good stretch, no matter what pose you're doing. Paradoxically, the more you can just enjoy each stretch, the faster you will progress. If you are in a hurry and practice with one eye on the next pose, it will actually slow you down. Trust me!

PRONE BACK STRETCH

1. Placement. Lie face down on your mat or blanket. Stretch your arms overhead and rest your hands on the floor. Keep your toes pointed and the inner edges of your legs together.

2. Pose. Stretch and lengthen from the fingertips to the toes.

Benefits: Prone Back Stretch provides an overall stretch.

SALABHASANA

LOCUST POSE

1. Placement. Lie face down on your mat or blanket. Place your chin on your mat or blanket. Keep your toes pointed and your inner ankles and knees touching. Rest your arms alongside of your body, palms facing down.

2. Pose. Keep both hips on your mat or blanket and on an exhalation stretch out through your right leg and lift it a few inches. Soften your throat and stretch through the crown of your head. Hold for three even breaths. Release on an exhale. Rest. Realign your body if necessary, and repeat with your left leg. As your strength increases, hold longer on each side.

3. Pose. To practice with both legs at the same time, turn the palms to face the body and place the knuckles under the groins. Exhale and stretch out through both legs and lift them, with the feet together and the knees straight. Hold for three even breaths at first. As your strength increases, hold the pose longer. Those with weak lower backs should do the one-legged version for at least a month, or until their strength has increased, before attempting this pose with two legs.

Caution: Those with disc problems should avoid this pose. Practice the first four poses in Chapter 12, "Relief: Back Stretches."

Benefits: Locust Pose (Salabhasana) strengthens the muscles of the lower back.

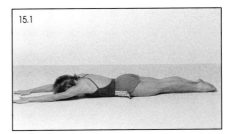

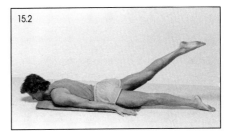

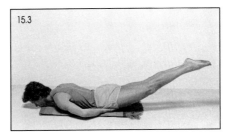

15.1 Prone Back Stretch
15.2 Locust Pose–single leg lift
15.3 Locust Pose–both legs lifted

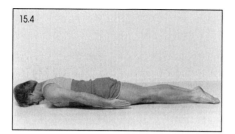

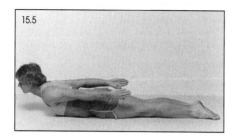

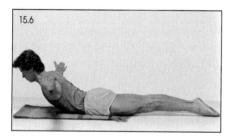

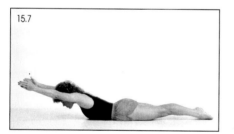

15.4   Preparation for Cobra
        Pose–placement
15.5   Preparation for Cobra
        Pose–arms extended back
15.6   Preparation for Cobra
        Pose–arms to sides
15.7   Preparation for Cobra
        Pose–arms overhead

BHUJANGASANA

PREPARATION FOR COBRA POSE

1. Placement. Lie face down on your mat or blanket. Place your forehead on your mat or blanket and your arms at your sides, palms facing in. Keep the inner edges of your legs and feet together and your toes pointing away.

2. Pose. Stretching out through your feet and legs, inhale and lift your head and upper chest. As you arch the back, remember to lengthen the front of the spine. Reach your hands back toward your feet. Press up through the crown of your head and look forward, keeping your throat soft. Hold for three even breaths. To release, gently lower your torso and rest your forehead on your mat or blanket. Gradually increase your time in the pose.

3. Variation. Practice as in #2, but change your arm positions. First, stretch the arms straight out from the shoulders. Second, place your arms overhead on your mat or blanket before lifting your head and chest. In all three ways of doing the pose, it is important that the breath be even, neither forced nor held. Holding the breath may lift you a fraction higher, but will drain you of energy.

Caution: Those with disc problems should avoid this pose. Practice the first four poses in Chapter 12, "Relief: Back Stretches."

Benefits: Preparation for Cobra Pose (Bhujangasana) strengthens the upper back muscles. Anyone who tends to have rounded shoulders should do this pose frequently—at least two or three times a week.

SUPPORTED CHEST OPENER

1. Placement. Make a roll with a firm blanket. Start small; you can always increase the size. Position the roll so that when you lie over it, the roll is behind the sternum (breastbone). Lean back on your elbows, and draw your chin in as you stretch your back over the roll and place your head on the floor. Straighten your legs out in front of you. Stretch your arms overhead. If your shoulders are tight and your arms don't touch the floor, support your forearms or hands with another blanket roll.

2. Pose. Draw the shoulder blades down the back, and the shoulders away from the ears. Stretch by extending through the heels and reaching through the fingertips. Soften your throat. Hold for one minute. Over time work up to three to four minutes.

3. Variation. If your neck feels uncomfortable or overarched, place a small folded towel under your head.

4. Variation. After you have given yourself a good stretch, you can just relax into the pose, enjoying the stretch created by letting go. Hold for up to five minutes. Be gentle!

Caution: If you feel discomfort in your lower back, bend your knees and place your feet on the floor. If your neck hurts, discontinue practice of this pose until you consult with a qualified teacher.

Benefits: Supported Chest Opener opens the chest and lengthens the spine.

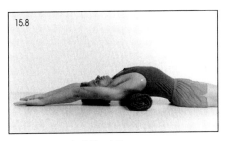

15.8   Supported Chest Opener

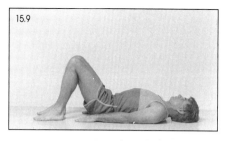

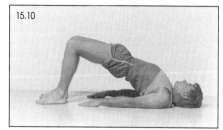

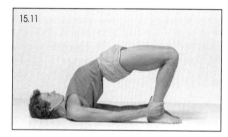

15.9   Bridge Pose–placement
15.10 Bridge Pose
15.11 Bridge Pose–holding ankles

SETU BANDHASANA

BRIDGE POSE

1. Placement. Sit on the floor, with your knees bent and your feet on the floor. Lean back on your elbows, and as you lie back stretch each vertebra away from the one below it. Place your shoulders and upper arms on a firmly folded blanket. Roll your shoulders back and down, and place your arms along the sides of your body, palms down. Lift the head and move the base of the skull away from the shoulders as you place the head back on the floor. Keep your throat soft and your face parallel to the ceiling. Keep your feet parallel to each other, in line with the outsides of your hips.

2. Pose. Exhale, press your feet firmly into the floor as you lift your pelvis. Lengthen the outer thighs toward the knees and the inner thighs toward the torso. From two inches below the navel, move the pubic bone down, and from above that spot, stretch the spine up toward the head. Let the throat rest back into the neck, and allow the back of the skull to stretch away from the shoulders. (This pose may also be done with the hands interlaced, stretching away from the head.) To release, gently roll your upper back and then your lumbar and then your pelvis to the floor. Imagine creating space between the vertebrae as the back is placed down.

3. Variation. Begin as in #1 and take hold of the ankles with the corresponding hands. (If you cannot reach your ankles, place a strap around your ankles, holding the strap with your arms extended.) Proceed as in #2, and roll the shoulders under to open the chest. Relax the face and throat, and allow the back of the skull to stretch away from the shoulders.

Benefits: In addition to the benefits of backbending, Bridge Pose (Setu Bandhasana) strengthens the knees. It also is an excellent preparation for Shoulderstand (Chapter 16).

USTRASANA

CAMEL POSE

1. Placement. Kneel and separate your legs hips' width apart. Place your hands at the sides of your hips. From the spot two inches below your navel, gently lengthen your pubic bone down. In this upright position keep your sternum (breastbone) aligned directly over your navel. Roll your shoulders back and down, and stretch up through the crown of your head.

2. Pose. Draw back with your thighs and let your pelvis pivot on your hip sockets as you arch your back and place one hand at a time on the heel or sole of each foot. Lengthen the front of the spine as it curves backward. Draw the chin in and then allow the head to drop back. Soften the front of the body. Keep the fronts of the ankles gently pressing into the floor, as this action naturally activates the thighs and thereby supports the pelvis. Stretch and enjoy. To release, pivot the pelvis on the hip sockets as you come upright, softening the fronts of the groins. Some people draw the chin toward the chest before they release the pose. Experiment and do what feels right for you.

3. Aid. To learn to bring your head back, sit on a chair and place your sitting bones far back on the seat. Lean forward slightly, lengthen your spine, and then lean into the back of the chair. Moving the tips of the shoulder blades down and the back of the head up, cup the head in the hands and slowly arch over the chair. Let the hands support and guide the head. Slowly return to an upright position, holding your head through the entire movement.

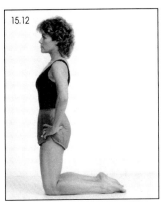

15.12

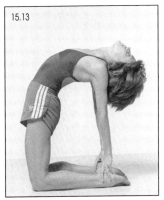

15.13

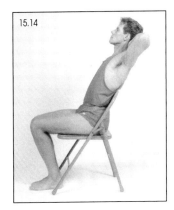

15.14

15.12 Camel Pose–placement
15.13 Camel Pose
15.14 Camel Pose–sitting on chair

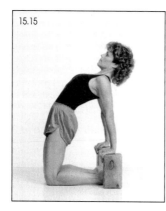

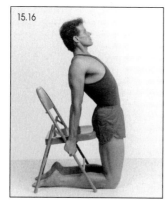

15.15   Camel Pose–with blocks
15.16   Camel Pose–hands on chair

4. Aid. Place a block (or two sturdy books identical in size) next to each ankle, and place your hands on them for support. Practice as in #2. Pay close attention to keeping the thighs active. The more you press down with the ankles, the more the spine will be able to stretch. (Again, for every action there is an opposite and equal reaction.)

5. Aid. Kneel with your back to a chair and place your palms on the seat of the chair, with your elbows drawn back and down. Practice as in #2. Pay close attention to keeping the thighs active. The more you gently press your ankles into the floor and your palms onto the seat of the chair, the more the spine will lengthen.

Caution: Those with neck problems should consult a qualified yoga teacher before practicing this pose.

Benefits: Camel Pose (Ustrasana) is very beneficial for those with rounded shoulders, who should practice this pose often. It opens the chest and brings mobility to the spine.

DHANURASANA

BOW POSE

1. Placement. Lie face down on your mat or blanket. Lengthen the front of your body, keeping the inner edges of your legs and feet touching. Exhale and bring the heels toward the buttocks. Your knees can separate, but keep the thighbones parallel. Reach back with your arms, and hold your right ankle with your right hand and your left ankle with your left hand.

2. Pose. Exhale and lift your torso and legs. Draw your legs away from your head as though reaching for the ceiling with your feet. Keep your arms lengthening, your throat relaxed, and your gaze soft. Firm the buttocks and lengthen from the groins to the knees. Keep the thighs parallel. Hold for fifteen seconds, breathing evenly. To release, lower your torso and thighs to your mat or blanket, release your feet, and lower your legs and forehead to your mat or blanket. Rest until the breath becomes quiet.

3. Variation. Inhale and practice with the thighs on the floor as you draw the feet away from the head. Lift your head and chest high off the floor. Keep your shoulders drawn down from your ears. Relax your abdomen, neck, and throat. Soften the stomach, relax the neck, and look straight ahead. Hold for two complete breaths. Gradually increase your time in the pose.

4. Aid. If you cannot reach your ankles or if your lower back feels pinched or compressed in this pose, you may need to practice with a strap around your ankles. Likewise, if you experience pain in the knees, holding a strap with the hands a few inches from the ankles may bring relief. After placing the strap around your ankles, proceed as in #2. Remember to firm the buttocks and lengthen from the groins to the knees. Always visualize making more space as you stretch.

Benefits: Bow Pose (Dhanurasana) brings elasticity and strength to the spine. It also stretches the groins.

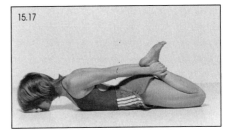

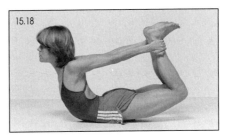

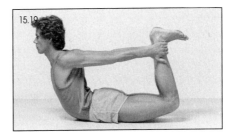

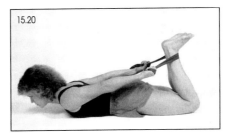

15.17   Bow Pose–placement
15.18   Bow Pose
15.19   Bow Pose–thighs on floor
15.20   Bow Pose–strap around
          ankles

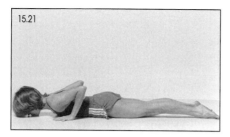

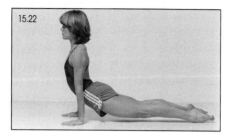

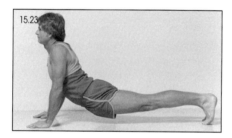

15.21 Upward-Facing Dog
Pose–placement
15.22 Upward-Facing Dog
Pose–on top of feet
15.23 Upward-Facing Dog
Pose–toes turned under

URDHVA MUKHA SVANASANA

UPWARD-FACING DOG POSE

1. Placement. Lie face down on your mat or blanket. Place your hands next to your chest, palms down, with your fingers facing forward. Keep your elbows in toward your body and pointing toward the ceiling. Separate your feet so they are hips' width apart. Rest on the tops of your feet. Lift the kneecaps to elongate the legs.

2. Pose. Inhale, straighten your arms, and lift your body so you are supported by your hands and the tops of your feet only. On an exhalation press the feet and hands down, draw the bottom tips of the shoulder blades down, and stretch out through the crown of the head. Look forward, keeping your gaze soft and your throat relaxed. Soften the front of the body and visualize the spine elongating. Hold for two complete breaths. Gradually increase your time in the pose to ten to fifteen seconds, breathing evenly. To release, gently lower your body, bring your hands to your sides, and rest your forehead on the floor.

3. Variation. Beginners should practice as in #2, but instead of resting on the tops of the feet, turn the toes under. Broaden the collarbones and lower the shoulders away from the ears. Be gentle and curious. Although this strengthens the arms, this pose is intended to stretch the spine. Let your spine extend backward and use your arms as support. Do not force the pose.

Benefits: Upward-Facing Dog Pose (Urdhva Mukha Svanasana) brings flexibility to the spine and blood to the pelvic region.

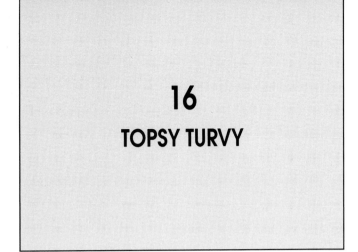

16
TOPSY TURVY

INVERTED POSES

Because gravity is an invisible force, few of us realize its effects on us. But even if we are not aware of gravity, we can witness these effects. The next time you're in the market, observe those around you. The power of gravity is reflected in sagging faces, breasts, bellies, and spines. The bones themselves are often misshapen by the compensations made in the effort to stay upright. Yogis have dealt with the effects of gravity for centuries. They have put gravity to good use by simply inverting the body for some time every day.

When the body is turned upside down, the organs in the abdominal cavity no longer weigh down on the pelvis. Body fluids are stimulated to move, and greater circulation is brought to different parts of the body. As this happens there is a greater exchange of fluids in each cell, nutrients are absorbed, and wastes are discarded more efficiently. With gravity's help the brain is flushed with blood and life-giving oxygen; the pituitary gland in the head and the thyroid and parathyroid glands in the neck are nourished. The venous blood in the lower body flows more freely toward the heart. Elimination is stimulated.

Elevating the legs after strenuous exercise is extremely important. Most athletic activities concentrate the flow of blood in the lower limbs. Unless this is reversed, the legs may feel heavy and the brain and heart may feel sluggish. Shoulderstand (Salamba Sarvangasana) and any of its variations can remedy these effects in minutes. This pose can be particularly beneficial if you work out in the morning and then sit or stand most of the rest of the day. If you have been running for more than a half hour, wait at least as long as you ran before elevating the legs. Otherwise, too much blood may flush the heart.

Things You Need To Know Before Practicing Shoulderstand

In Shoulderstand the musculature of the arms, shoulders, and neck are strengthened. In addition, the lower back, abdomen, and leg muscles are toned by the essential work of balancing upside down. This pose is one of total equilibrium. As in all poses, the entire body must coordinate its efforts to do the pose properly.

The vertebrae of the neck are much smaller than the rest of the spine; they are not designed to bear a lot of weight. To prevent injury, do not press the back of the neck into the floor. To preserve the concave curve of the neck most of us need to work with the shoulders raised slightly higher than the back of the head. To do this, place two folded blankets (or more if necessary), each about one or two inches thick, under your shoulders and arms. The back of your head rests on the floor, and the back of your neck is still in its natural concave curve, gently arching into your body.

In Shoulderstand the back of the neck will be lengthening, so expect the feeling of stretch. To protect the neck, never turn the head from side to side in Shoulderstand (or Plough Pose). If the neck hurts or the throat feels compressed, very gently lift the chin a half inch or so, and relax the neck, throat, and face. Or you might lift the shoulders still higher by placing more blankets under them. If you feel strain in the neck, however, come down. Practice a modified version of the pose; for example, use chairs or the wall. If you still have problems, consult with a qualified yoga teacher.

Beginners may sometimes feel discomfort in the neck or lower back after doing inverted poses. For relief, do the Knees-to-Chest Pose, #3 (Chapter 12). Lift the head to the knees three or four times or until the discomfort is gone.

Although you may not believe it at first, Shoulderstand has a soothing effect on the nerves and acts to bring about relaxation. If you run or work out at night and find that this stimulates you so much that you have insomnia, five to ten minutes of Shoulderstand will help you fall asleep. But no matter when you choose to do this pose, be sure to do it. Soon you won't have to be told about the benefits of inverting the body, because they will be yours.

Caution: Those with high blood pressure, a detached retina, or glaucoma should not do these poses without the guidance of a qualified teacher.

For women: During the active bleeding phase of your menstrual period (the first four or five days or the second through the fifth days—whenever the flow is heaviest), do not invert the body.

NECK STRETCH

1. Placement. Lie on your back in Mountain Pose. Bend your knees and place your feet on the floor near your buttocks. Interlace your fingers behind your head.

2. Pose. Exhale, and with the neck and head completely passive, lift the head with the hands. Bring your head as far forward as possible without strain. Draw your shoulders away from your ears.

Benefits: Neck Stretch stretches and relieves tension in the neck and upper shoulders. It also prepares you for Shoulderstand or Plough Pose.

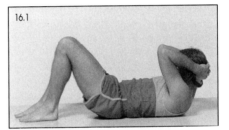

16.1   Neck Stretch–head passive

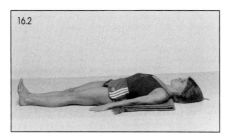

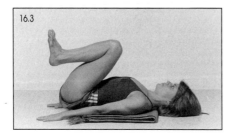

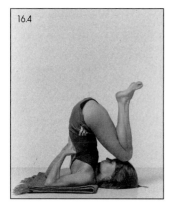

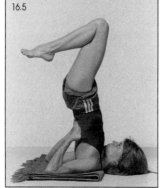

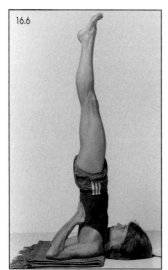

16.2   Shoulderstand–placement
        on blanket
16.3   Shoulderstand–knees to
        chest
16.4   Shoulderstand–on shoulders,
        knees to head
16.5   Shoulderstand–knees lifted
16.6   Shoulderstand

SALAMBA SARVANGASANA

SHOULDERSTAND

1. Placement. Lie in Mountain Pose, with your shoulders at the edge of two or more folded blankets. Roll your shoulders toward the floor to open your chest. Place your hands on the floor, palms facing down, and with an exhalation, bend your knees and bring your legs over your chest.

2. Pose. Exhale, press the hands into the floor, firm the lower abdomen, and lift the buttocks toward the ceiling. Bend your arms and place your palms on your back, as close to the floor as possible. Keep your fingers pointing toward the ceiling if possible. Exhale and lift your knees toward the ceiling. Straighten both legs, keeping the thighs active throughout the pose. Let your inner feet and legs touch. Exhale and lengthen from the shoulders to the elbows, pressing the upper arms into the floor to lift the entire body upward. Press the balls of the feet toward the ceiling, but keep the groins soft. Allow your neck, face, and throat to be passive. Hold for twenty to thirty seconds, breathing evenly. Gradually increase your time in the pose to five minutes. Don't be in a hurry to do this; allow your practice to build. To release, bend your legs and bring your knees to your head and your hands to the floor. Slowly roll the back and legs to the floor, keeping the head on the floor throughout.

3. Variation. In the beginning you may not have the flexibility to lift high and onto the tops of the shoulders. If this is the case, place your hands on your back closer to your buttocks. The legs will be at an angle, over your head. As your flexibility and strength increase, work toward lifting the body until it is perpendicular to the floor.

4. Aid. Lie with your buttocks against a wall. Stretch your legs up the wall (see Staff Pose, Chapter 17). Bend your legs and place your feet on the wall. Exhale and press the feet into the wall. On your next exhalation, begin lifting your pelvis until you are on the tops of your shoulders. Interlace your fingers and stretch your hands toward the wall and down to the floor. Keeping your elbows close to each other, release your hands and place them on your back as close to the floor as possible. Practice this version of Shoulderstand every day for a week. Then practice lifting one foot from the wall, placing that foot back on the wall, and lifting the other one. Do this every day for a week. With this type of cautious preparation you may be ready to take both feet off the wall. (If not, continue with this modified version until you can safely and confidently do so.) Take one leg away from the wall at a time and then straighten both legs. Hold for fifteen to twenty seconds, breathing evenly. To release, place one foot at a time back on the wall and roll down slowly.

Benefits: Shoulderstand (Salamba Sarvangasana) relieves fatigue, calms and rejuvenates the body, strengthens the upper body, and stretches the neck.

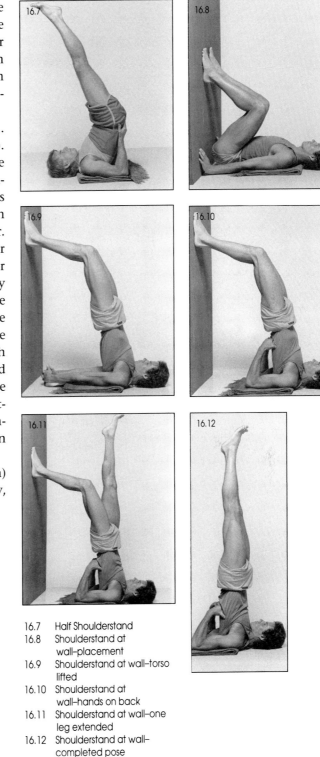

16.7 Half Shoulderstand
16.8 Shoulderstand at wall–placement
16.9 Shoulderstand at wall–torso lifted
16.10 Shoulderstand at wall–hands on back
16.11 Shoulderstand at wall–one leg extended
16.12 Shoulderstand at wall–completed pose

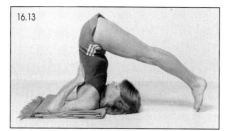

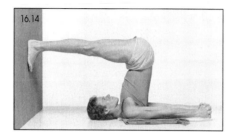

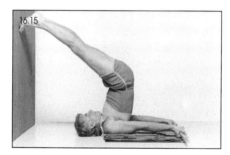

16.13 Plough Pose
16.14 Plough Pose–fingers inter-
       laced
16.15 Plough Pose–holding a pole

HALASANA

PLOUGH POSE

1. Placement. Begin in Shoulderstand.

2. Pose. Exhale and, lifting your sitting bones up, lower your legs overhead until the tips of your toes touch the floor. Keep your feet perpendicular to the floor. Stretch your pubic bone away from your sternum, which will enable your spine to lengthen and not collapse. Keep your thighs active, and keep your face, neck, and abdomen passive. Hold for ten to fifteen seconds. Gradually increase your time in the pose to one to two minutes. To release, place the hands on the floor, and roll one vertebra at a time to the floor. Plough Pose is traditionally practiced before coming out of Shoulderstand and for half of the time Shoulderstand is held. It can also be used as a therapeutic pose to rest and rehabilitate the nervous system, as in #6.

3. Variation. Come into Plough Pose. Interlace your fingers as you straighten your arms and stretch them down to the floor and away from your body. This opens the chest and stretches the shoulders and arms.

4. Aid. If the arms, shoulders, or chest are tight you may not be able to interlace the fingers behind you. In that case, hold a pole or towel in your hands, straighten your arms, and stretch your arms down to the floor. As your flexibility increases, move your hands closer and closer to each other. Discard the aid when you are able to clasp your hands.

5. Aid. Lie on your back on your blanket with the top of your head toward a wall. Stretch your arms overhead and place yourself so that your outstretched fingers are one or two inches away from the wall. Then lower your arms to your sides. Come into Shoulderstand and place your hands on your back. To come into Plough Pose, exhale and lower both legs overhead until your feet are on the wall. If your hamstrings are tight, your feet will be higher up the wall. If the hamstrings are stretched, the legs will be horizontal or even closer to the floor. No matter where your feet are, keep your thighs active and lift your sitting bones. Relax your face, neck, and abdomen.

6. Aid. Plough Pose, when done with a chair, is a marvelous resting pose and is soothing to the nervous system. It is also helpful in relieving headaches. Place the back of a folding chair against a wall. Lie on one or more blankets in Mountain Pose, with the top of your head facing the chair. Come into Shoulderstand with your legs bent. Reach overhead and pull the chair in so it is close to your head. Bend your knees and place them on the seat of the chair, resting your lower legs against the back of the chair. Rest your arms on the floor, either behind your back or overhead. Once you are familiar with this version of Plough Pose, you can rest in this position for up to ten minutes. To release, bring your arms overhead and push the chair back against the wall. Then with bent knees and hands on the floor, slowly lower your torso and legs down to the floor.

Benefits: Plough Pose (Halasana) gives you the same benefits as Shoulderstand. In addition, it stretches the legs and strengthens the back.

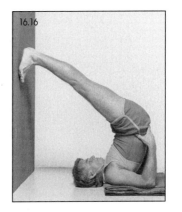

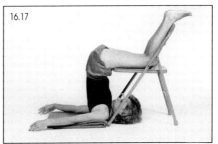

16.16   Plough Pose–feet on wall
16.17   Plough Pose–knees on chair

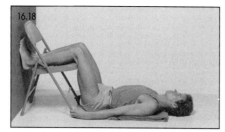

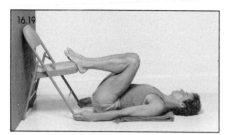

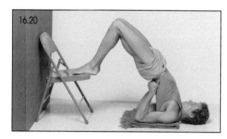

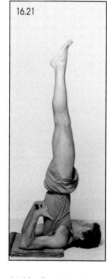

16.18 Shoulderstand with chair–placement
16.19 Shoulderstand with chair–feet on chair
16.20 Shoulderstand with chair–torso lifted
16.21 Shoulderstand with chair–completed pose

SALAMBA SARVANGASANA AND HALASANA

SHOULDERSTAND AND PLOUGH POSE WITH CHAIRS

This variation of Shoulderstand and Plough Pose has several stages. Read these instructions all the way through at least once before proceeding.

1. Placement. Place the back of a sturdy chair against a wall. Then position a folded blanket so that when you lie with your shoulders on it, your buttocks are in line with the front edge of the chair and your lower legs rest on the seat. Place a second chair behind you and far enough away so that when you lower your legs from Shoulderstand to Plough Pose your feet will rest on the second chair. Remember that when you come into Shoulderstand and Plough Pose the head remains on the floor and the neck lengthens, but does not press down into the mat or the floor.

2. Preparation. Bend your legs and place your feet on the edge of the seat. Exhale, press the feet into the chair, and lift the torso high. Interlace your fingers and stretch your arms toward the wall. Squeeze the shoulder blades toward each other and allow the chest to open. Relax your neck, throat, and face. Bring your hands to rest on your back.

3. Preparation. Exhale lift one leg up to the ceiling. On the next exhalation lift the other leg. Hold for a few breaths in Shoulderstand.

4. Preparation. Exhale, bend at the hips, and lower the legs into Plough Pose onto the chair behind you. Release your hands and hold the legs of the chair at your back. Move the chair toward you until it touches your back.

5. Pose. With your upper arms inside the front legs of the chair, hold the back legs of the chair near the seat. Use this as a lever to roll the armpits open. Rest in Plough Pose. Exhale and lift one leg at a time to the ceiling. Keep the chair touching the back as you continue to lift through the legs and feet. Eventually you will be high on your shoulders and your body will be vertical. To release, lower both legs back to Plough Pose. Move the chair at your back to one side, place your hands on the floor behind your back, and roll your back down, one vertebra at a time, keeping your head on the floor. When your legs are vertical, bend your knees to your chest, and place your feet on the floor.

Benefits: Shoulderstand (Salamba Sarvangasana) and Plough Pose (Halasana) with Chairs stretches the chest and shoulders. It teaches correct Shoulderstand alignment and helps build time in inverted poses.

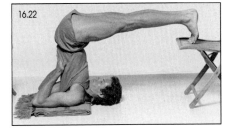

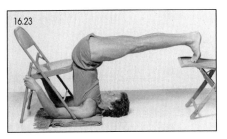

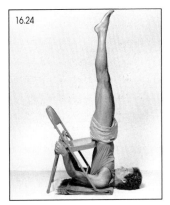

16.22 Plough Pose with chair–feet on chair
16.23 Plough Pose with chair–draw chair to support back
16.24 Shoulderstand with chair–chair supports back

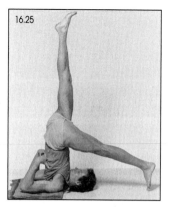

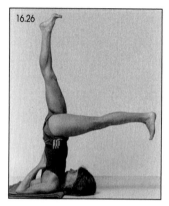

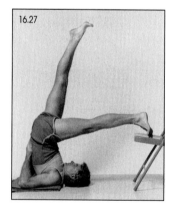

16.25 One-Legged Shoulderstand
16.26 One-Legged
      Shoulderstand–leg parallel
      to floor
16.27 One-Legged
      Shoulderstand–foot on chair

EKA PADA SARVANGASANA

ONE-LEGGED SHOULDERSTAND

1. Placement. Begin in Shoulderstand, with your hands placed on your back.

2. Pose. Look at the right foot and visually gauge where it is in relation to the ceiling. This helps you stay properly aligned in the pose. Without moving your right leg, lower your left leg to the floor. Keep both thighs active. Roll your right thigh in and lift your outer left hip. Release any tension in the face, neck, and throat. Hold for five to ten seconds. Exhale and lift your leg. Practice on the opposite side. Gradually increase your time on each side to thirty seconds.

3. Variation. Practice as in #2, but keep the left leg parallel to the floor (without taking the foot to the floor). Work on keeping the pelvic bones even while stretching the pubic bone toward the ceiling.

4. Aid. Practice with a chair behind your head so that in #3 your foot rests on a chair.

Benefits: One-Legged Shoulderstand (Eka Pada Sarvangasana) strengthens and stretches the legs and groins. It also massages the abdominal organs.

SUPTA KONASANA

OPEN ANGLE SHOULDERSTAND

1. Placement. Begin in Shoulderstand, with your hands on your back.

2. Pose. Exhale and open the legs to the sides. Keep your feet squared and your kneecaps lifted. As you lower your feet to the floor, lift your sitting bones toward the ceiling.

3. Variation. To rest, bend the legs and bring the soles of the feet together (as in Bound Angle Pose, Chapter 9). Keep your heels as close to your groins as possible.

Benefits: Open Angle Shoulderstand (Supta Konasana) rests the legs while building time in Shoulderstand. It also stretches the inner thighs and develops balance.

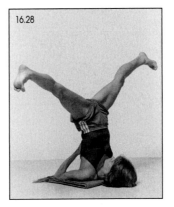

16.28

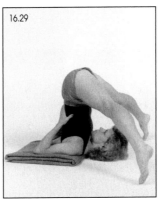

16.29

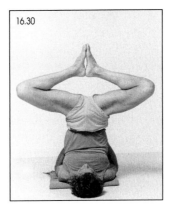

16.30

16.28 Open Angle
Shoulderstand–extend legs
to sides
16.29 Open Angle
Shoulderstand–feet on floor
16.30 Bound Angle Shoulderstand

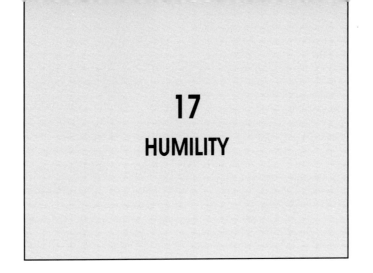

17
HUMILITY

SITTING FORWARD BENDS

The forward bending poses seem to capture the essential benefits of yoga: an elongated body that houses a quiet mind. They are extremely beneficial for athletes, because they stretch the entire back side of the body. These poses teach perseverance, patience, and surrender, because these qualities are required for their successful execution. While these poses are held, the complaining mind learns to surrender to the discomfort felt in the legs and in the back. This surrender can become a doorway to a quiet world within the body.

If you are a beginning student, however, forward bending may not be so quiet. The legs may immediately cry out. This is the reaction of the powerful hamstring muscles. (Postures for elongating these muscles are given in Chapter 10, "The Screamers: Hamstring Stretches.") The back is also given an intense stretch. It is essential to protect the back by doing forward bends in the correct manner. Staff Pose (Dandasana), although not a forward bend, is included in this chapter to aid you in understanding the proper and safe way in which to bend.

Visualize the body in Staff Pose as a pocketknife, with a blade opened to a 90-degree angle. The torso is the blade, the hips form the hinge, and the legs are the case. Allow the blade (the torso) to close slowly, bend-

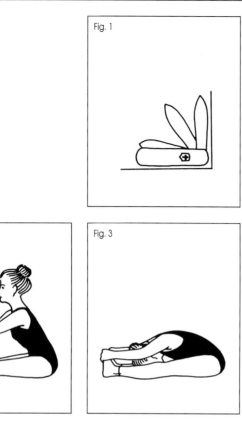

Fig. 1

Fig. 2

Fig. 3

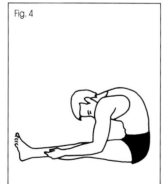

Fig. 4

Fig. 1   The principles of correct forward bending can be compared to a pocket knife.

Fig. 2   The torso is the blade, the hips form the hinge, and the legs are the case.

Fig. 3   Always bend from the hinge of the hips.

Fig. 4   In this incorrect forward bend, the pelvis is tilted back and the upper back is rounded.

ing from the hinge (the hips), and fitting neatly just inside the case (the legs). The trunk and legs are therefore in parallel planes. The arms come forward to hook the feet and to secure the position.

Let's examine the crucial factor in this closing movement: the efficiency of the bending point. In order for the body to stretch forward easily without damaging the back, several things must happen. The hamstrings, the calf muscles, and the muscles of the lower back must lengthen and the pelvis must be tipped forward. This pelvic tilt is most important. When you sit as far forward as possible on the sitting bones and continue to move these bones away from the knees, you guarantee the safety of the spine. The back will be long, like the straight edge of the knife's blade. If the forward bend is begun with the pelvis tilted back, as in the illustration, the legs are not stretched adequately, and the back is severely overstretched. This incorrect movement makes practicing the pose dangerous, instead of beneficial.

As you do Staff Pose and forward bends, keep the feet active and squared, so the inner edges of the feet are parallel with the outer edges. Doing Staff Pose with the feet against a wall will show you how to do this.

Perseverance is required to hold these poses, and patience is developed and nurtured in that holding. As the forward bends are held for increasingly longer periods, the mind may protest even more strongly against the discomfort. Eventually the mind learns to surrender to the poses. The surrender is developed only by many hours of practice, so do not be discouraged by the impatience that permeates your poses in the beginning.

Caution: When doing these poses, do not attempt to close the torso to the legs in the beginning stages of your practice. Simply come into the poses as far as you can with the spine fully extended.

DANDASANA
STAFF POSE

1. Placement. Sit on your sitting bones with your legs extended out in front of you and in line with your hips. If necessary, sit on one or more folded blankets. Keep your feet, hips, and shoulders in line and squared with a wall.

2. Pose. Keep your legs active and your spine lifting. The more you move the thighbones toward the floor, the more lift you will observe in the spine. Keep the kneecaps lifted. Place your palms (or fingertips) on the floor and in line with your hips. Press down with the hands to help lift the torso.

3. Aid. If it is difficult to maintain the lift of the spine, sit on the edge of a firmly folded blanket, and place a belt or tie around the balls of your feet. Hold the tie with both hands and with the arms extended. As before, press your thighbones down, and observe the lift that comes to the spine.

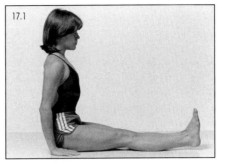

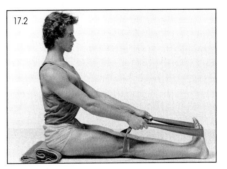

17.1   Staff Pose
17.2   Staff Pose–on blanket with
          belt

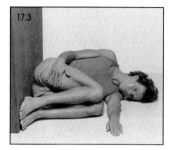

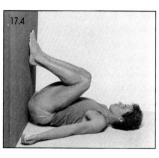

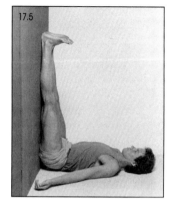

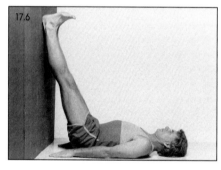

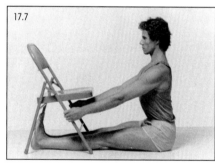

4. Aid. Do Staff Pose with your legs up the wall. Lie on your left side with your knees bent and your buttocks and feet touching the wall. Roll onto the back, keeping the knees bent. On an exhalation stretch your legs up the wall, keeping them straight. If your legs bend or your buttocks are off the floor, move back from the wall far enough to allow your legs to gently straighten and your buttocks to rest on the floor. (This is essential for bending at the crease between the legs and torso. Otherwise you are bending from the spine and therefore straining the back.) Square the feet and lengthen the pubic bone toward the wall. Keep your shoulders low, away from your ears, and your palms flat on the floor (or on the wall). Sometimes work in this pose by pausing on an inhalation, and on an exhalation stretching the legs while you lengthen the pubic bone. Sometimes rest in this pose, noticing where you are tight on an inhalation, and letting go on an exhalation. To come down, bend your knees and place your feet flat on the wall. Roll to one side and sit up.

5. Aid. Sit on the floor opposite a folding chair. Place your feet against the back rung of the chair, as pictured. Hold the seat of the chair with the hands, dropping the thighbones and lifting the spine with each exhalation.

Caution: Understanding this pose is essential before proceeding to the forward bends. If the vertebrae of the lower back protrude in Staff Pose, then do all the following sitting poses with a folded blanket under your buttocks. The prop should be high enough to tilt the pelvis slightly forward and maintain the lift of the lower back.

Benefits: Staff Pose (Dandasana) elongates and strengthens the front body and back body equally. It also stretches the legs.

17.3　Staff Pose–buttocks to wall
17.4　Staff Pose at wall–roll onto back
17.5　Staff Pose at wall–legs extended
17.6　Staff Pose at wall–for tight hamstrings
17.7　Staff Pose–with chair

JANU SIRSASANA

HEAD-TO-KNEE POSE

1. Placement. Sit in Staff Pose. Bend the right leg, bringing the heel toward the right sitting bone. Let the right leg drop to the side so it rests on the outer thigh and knee. Keep your left leg extended and turned slightly in.

2. Pose. Inhale and raise both arms overhead. Feel the lift originating from the sides of the abdomen. Exhale and bend forward from your hips. Rest the sternum on the knee and the chin on the shin. The vertical lift of the torso has now become horizontal. Hold first the toes of your extended foot, and over time gradually extend your stretch to catch your sole, eventually holding your wrists beyond your foot. Hold for a few breaths. Release and repeat for an equal number of breaths on the opposite side.

3. Variation. Practice as in #2, but do not take the torso down this time. Reach your arms forward and hold the outer edges of your feet. Work on achieving length of the spine by stretching the pubic bone down and pressing out through the crown of the head.

4. Aid. Place a folded towel or blanket under your bent knee if it does not touch the floor. Use a tie around the foot of the extended leg, holding an end in each hand. Remain sitting upright, using the props to help you open the hip and lengthen the spine. Hold for four or five even breaths. Practice on the opposite side.

Benefits: Head-to-Knee Pose (Janu Sirsasana) gives an intense stretch to the extended leg, opens the hips, tones and stimulates the internal organs, and strengthens and elongates the spine.

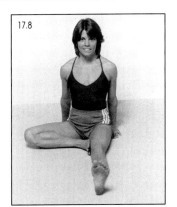

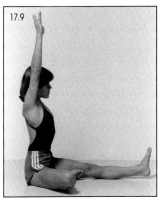

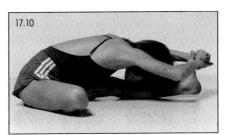

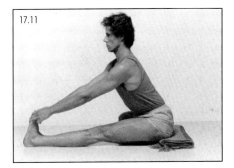

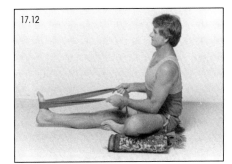

17.8   Head-to-Knee Pose–placement
17.9   Head-to-Knee Pose–arms overhead
17.10 Head-to-Knee Pose
17.11 Head-to-Knee Pose–with spine extended
17.12 Head-to-Knee Pose–with blanket and belt

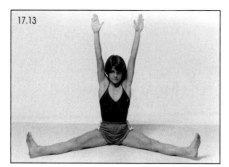

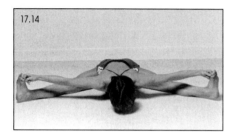

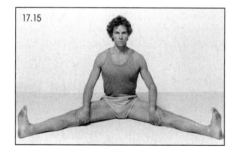

17.13 Open Angle Pose–
placement
17.14 Open Angle Pose
17.15 Open Angle Pose–holding
thighs

UPAVISTHA KONASANA

OPEN ANGLE POSE

1. Placement. Sit in Staff Pose. Spread your legs wide apart, keeping your legs active and your kneecaps facing the ceiling. Stretch the arms overhead and lengthen the spine. Allow the lift to come from the sides of the abdomen.

2. Pose. Exhale, lengthen the spine, and come forward to take hold of the big toes with the thumbs and next two fingers. Exhale, drop the thighbones, and bend from the hip crease, extending the front and back of your torso evenly toward the floor. Eventually your chest and chin will come to rest on the floor. Hold for a few even breaths, gradually increasing your time in the pose to one minute. Come up on an inhalation and return to Staff Pose.

3. Variation. Practice as in #1, but hold the insides of your thighs with your fingers under your thighs and your elbows bent. Drop your elbows back, using your arms to lift and extend your spine. Your torso remains in Staff Pose, with your shoulders moving down and back.

4. Aid. Wrap a tie around each foot, and hold the ends of the tie with your arms extended. Do not come forward, but use the ties to help you lengthen the spine. If your spine is collapsed, sit on the edge of a folded blanket.

5. Aid. Another very useful way to practice this pose is with the legs up the wall. Stretch your legs up the wall in Staff Pose, as described earlier in this chapter. Then allow your legs to spread apart, but keep your feet squared. Allow gravity to slowly lengthen the inner thighs. To increase the stretch, place your hands on your inner thighs and gently press your legs toward the floor.

Caution: If you feel pain in the inner knees in this pose, bring the legs closer together. If the pain persists, consult a teacher.

Benefits: Open Angle Pose (Upavistha Konasana) stretches the inner legs and opens the groins and hips. It is of special benefit to women, because it improves circulation to the female reproductive organs.

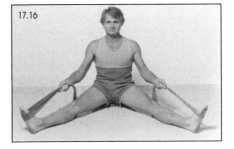

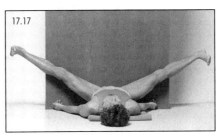

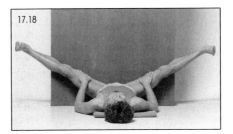

17.16 Open Angle Pose–on blanket with belts
17.17 Open Angle Pose–lying at wall
17.18 Open Angle Pose–at wall pressing thighs

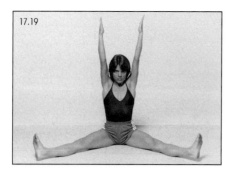

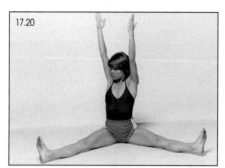

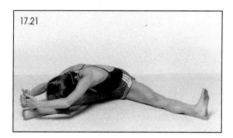

PARSVA UPAVISTHA KONASANA
SIDE VARIATION OF OPEN ANGLE POSE

1. Placement. Begin in Staff Pose, and spread your legs wide apart. Lifting one buttock at a time, move the flesh of the buttocks back with the hands so you feel the contact of the sitting bones with the floor or blanket. Inhale and lift your arms overhead.

2. Pose. Exhale, turn your torso to the right, keeping your legs in the placement position. Exhale, stretch forward from your hip joints, and rest your torso on your right leg. Encourage both thighbones to drop toward the floor. Take hold of your foot as in Head-to-Knee Pose. Hold for a few breaths. To come up, stretch your arms out in front of you and raise your arms and torso as a single unit. Come back to center, and then practice to the opposite side.

17.19   Side Variation of Open
           Angle Pose–placement
17.20   Side Variation of Open
           Angle Pose–torso rotated
17.21   Side Variation of Open
           Angle Pose

3. Variation. Practice as in #1, and rotate your trunk to the right. Take hold of your right foot with both hands. On an inhalation allow your thighbones to drop, your collarbones to broaden, and your spine to lengthen. On an exhalation, move your elongated spine slightly forward, stretching your pubic bone down. Work gently in this manner for several breaths. Do not disturb the position of your left foot. Release and practice to the opposite side.

4. Aid. Sit on a firmly folded blanket. Place a tie around your right foot. Use the tie to help you lengthen your torso. Then work as in #3.

Benefits: Side Variation of Open Angle Pose (Parsva Upavistha Konasana) stretches the inner thighs, groins, and hips. In addition, both sides of the torso are given an intense stretch.

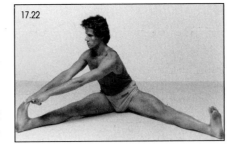

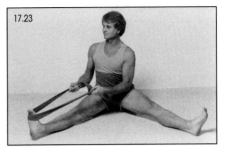

17.22 Side Variation of Open
Angle Pose–extending spine
17.23 Side Variation of Open
Angle Pose–on blanket
with tie

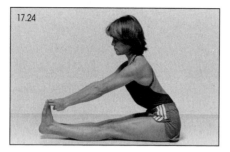

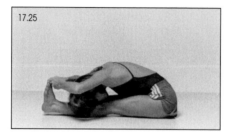

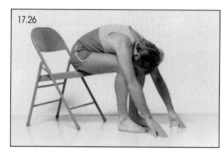

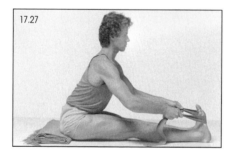

17.24 Seated Forward
Bend–extending spine
17.25 Seated Forward Bend
17.26 Seated Forward Bend–
on chair
17.27 Seated Forward Bend–
on blanket with tie

PASCHIMOTTANASANA

SEATED FORWARD BEND

1. Placement. Begin in Staff Pose. Inhale and raise your arms overhead. Remember that the lift of the arms begins at the sides of the abdomen.

2. Pose. Exhale and, bending from your hips, extend your torso over your legs and take hold of your big toes. You will eventually be able to rest your entire torso and head on your legs. Hold for a few breaths as you stretch both sides of the torso evenly, over time working up to one minute. Exhale, drop the thighs down, and stretch the pubic bone away from the breastbone. Inhale, stretch your arms out in front of you, and, lifting your arms and torso as a single unit, come back to an upright position. Bring your arms down to your sides and sit in Staff Pose.

3. Variation. Place the back of a chair against a wall. Sit on the edge of the chair seat with your knees bent and your feet on the floor. Separate your feet so they are hips' width apart. Inhale and raise your arms overhead, as in #1. Exhale, bend from your hips, and extend your arms and torso forward. Let your arms hang loosely at your sides. Remain in this position for several breaths, allowing the spine to lengthen and the muscles of the back to release.

4. Aid. Practice Staff Pose, sitting on a folded blanket. Your lift should be high enough to allow you to maintain the lumbar curve. Place a strap or towel around the balls of your feet. On an exhalation bend your elbows and move your breastbone toward your toes. Remember to bend from your hips.

Benefits: Seated Forward Bend (Paschimottanasana) gives an intense stretch to the back of the body and massages the abdominal organs. When done correctly, it is a calming pose.

18
REVOLVE AND RESOLVE

TWISTING POSES

For many people the word *yoga* evokes images of pretzel-shaped bodies knotted into impossible twists. A Western misunderstanding of yoga and a general misconception of the purpose of the poses have led to this confusion.

Sometimes a student comes to yoga class with a desire to realize this contorted image with his or her own body. This student is disappointed to learn that the twisting poses are not designed to create human pretzels. Twists are neither casually slipped into nor aggressively forced. They are done with the same precision and awareness that is demanded by all of the postures.

But twisting poses are not the exclusive domain of the experienced or more flexible student. Presented here are those twists that are both possible to practice as well as beneficial for the beginner. They also form the foundation for more advanced twists. They can be especially useful in a yoga practice before or after athletic competition because of their tension-relieving effects.

The essential principle of twisting poses is that the spine must be lengthened as it turns. Visualize a spiral and create space between the vertebrae as you twist. Elongate the front and back of the torso evenly to create a shallow indentation where the spine lies. Let your torso be long and graceful; resist any notion of hurry or

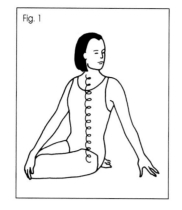

Fig. 1

Fig. 1   Twist by extending the spine, then turning. Visualize the spine making a spiral motion, one vertebra turning above the other.

forcing. This way your spine will begin to feel like a spiral of gossamer thread that is growing longer and longer. If you force yourself, the experience will be more like a thick wire mattress coil compressed to support a two hundred-pound weight.

There are two simple ways to check the extension of the spine. One is to see if the shoulders are horizontal. Unevenness here indicates one side or other of the spine is compressed. Now and then practice in front of a mirror to check whether your shoulders are even. The second way to check for spinal extension in twists is to touch your spine at the waist to see if the spine is indented here. If the vertebrae poke out, continue to lengthen the pubic bone down or work with the variations and aids described for each pose (or do both).

As you twist, turn the flesh of the lower abdomen in the direction your shoulders are turning. This action stimulates twisting from the base of the spine and tones the abdominal area. Also, never lead the twisting motion with the head. Simply allow the head to follow the direction of the twist. If you lead with your head, neck strain and discomfort can result.

Caution: People with medically diagnosed herniated discs should practice only the Chair Twist until the condition improves. Practice instead standing poses (no twists), back stretches, and gentle backbends.

CHAIR TWIST

1. Placement. Place the back of a sturdy chair, preferably a folding chair, against a wall. Sit on the edge of the chair, with your feet parallel on the floor and slightly apart. Sit forward on the sitting bones and lengthen the spine. Draw your shoulders down from your ears, and check that your chin is parallel to the floor.

2. Pose. Exhale, stretch your left hand behind you as far as possible onto the back of the chair, and with your right hand hold the back of the chair. Keep both elbows pointing down and the collarbones broad. On an exhalation, continue walking your fingers to the left as you elongate your spine and turn. Keep your feet even on the floor. Gently turn your navel to the left. Hold for fifteen seconds, breathing evenly. Release slowly and come back to center. Allow the breath to return to normal and practice on the opposite side.

3. Variation. Sit sideways on the chair so that the left side of your body is facing the wall. Be sure to sit forward on the sitting bones. Secure your left leg against the back of the chair as shown. Inhale and lengthen your spine; exhale and turn to the left and hold the chair back with both hands. Pause with each inhalation, and stretch up and turn farther to the left with each exhalation. Draw the abdomen to the left. Push with the left hand, pull with the right hand. Keep the collarbones broad and the breath soft.

4. Aid. If your feet don't reach the floor, use two thick books under your feet to enable you to keep your heels down.

Benefits: Chair Twist teaches the principle of extension during a twisting movement. It also releases tension in the spine.

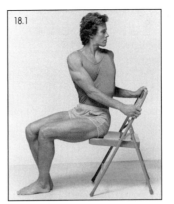

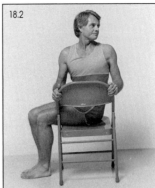

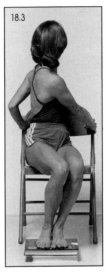

18.1   Chair Twist–back to chair
18.2   Chair Twist–side to chair
18.3   Chair Twist–feet supported

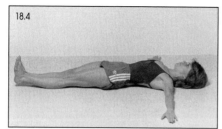

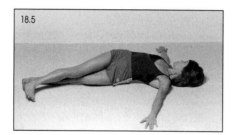

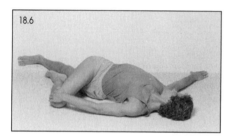

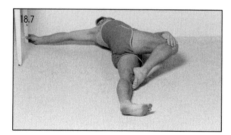

18.4   Crocodile Twist–placement
18.5   Crocodile Twist–heel on toes
18.6   Crocodile Twist–arch to
        knee
18.7   Crocodile Twist–holding
        anchor

CROCODILE TWIST

1. Placement. Lie on your back in Mountain Pose. Extend your arms out at shoulder level so you form a T position. Turn your palms down.

2. Pose. Exhale and extend out through your heels. Lift the right foot, wedging the right heel between the left big toe and the second toe. Exhale and roll the feet to the left without disturbing the position of the right foot. Allow your right hip to roll to the left, drawing your left hip under you. Keep both shoulders on the floor, and turn your head to look out over your right hand. On an exhalation turn your navel to the left. Hold for ten to fifteen seconds, breathing evenly. Release back to center and practice on the opposite side.

3. Variation. Place the arch of your right foot on top of your left knee, and bring your left hand onto your right knee. Exhale and, without disturbing your shoulders, shift onto the side of your left hip and lower your right knee to the left, as your turn your head to the right. Lengthen your pubic bone down. Pause on an inhalation and on an exhalation gently press the right knee toward the floor, turning the lower abdomen to the right, all the while extending from the left leg through the crown of the head. Release back to the center, realign your body in Mountain Pose, and practice on the other side. Do the pose at least twice on each side.

4. Aid. Practice near a sturdy piece of furniture (one that is not going to fall over on you), and use this as an anchor for your arm and shoulder. Hold onto the furniture as you turn the legs and hips in the opposite direction.

Benefits: Crocodile Twist massages and revitalizes the spine, and releases tension in the body.

JATHARA PARIVARTANASANA, VARIATION

FLOOR TWIST

1. Placement. Lie on your back in Mountain Pose. Extend your arms out at shoulder level so that your body forms a T position. With the tips of your shoulder blades drawn down, turn your palms down.

2. Pose. Exhale and with your pubic bone lengthening down, bend both legs and bring your knees to your chest. Exhale, roll to your right so that your right knee touches the floor. Turn the flesh of your lower abdomen away from your knees. Take a few breaths and repeat to the left. Bring your legs back to center and lower your feet to the floor. Then repeat the cycle again.

3. Variation. Beginning in Mountain Pose, lie on your back, bend your knees and bring your feet flat on the floor near your buttocks. Roll onto the sides of your feet and take your knees toward the floor to the left. On each exhalation, lengthen the right knee away from the torso and gently toward the floor. Also on each exhalation, turn the lower abdomen to the right. Hold the pose for five or six breaths and repeat to the opposite side. Practice the pose on each side two or three times.

4. Aid. Practice near a sturdy piece of furniture. Grasp it with the left hand, so that when you turn to the right, the left arm and shoulder receive a stretch. Then practice on the opposite side.

Caution: Do not do this pose if you have disc problems. Focus instead on spinal stretches and standing poses.

Benefits: Floor Twist (Preparation for Jathara Parivartanasana) relieves lower back pain caused by muscular tension and tones the abdominal area.

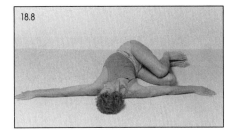

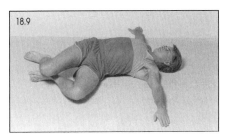

18.8   Floor Twist
18.9   Floor Twist–feet on floor

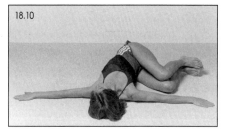

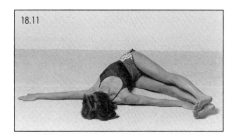

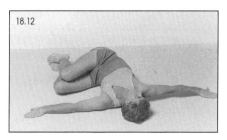

18.10 Belly Turning Pose–knees to side
18.11 Belly Turning Pose–straighten legs
18.12 Belly Turning Pose–feet on floor

JATHARA PARIVARTANASANA

BELLY TURNING POSE

1. Placement. Lie on your back in Mountain Pose. Take your arms out to your sides so that your body forms a T position. Turn your palms down.

2. Pose. Exhale and bend both legs, and bring both knees toward your chest. On your next exhalation take your knees to the right side and then straighten your legs. Keep your thighs active and lengthen through your heels as you bring your feet toward your right hand. Keep the left shoulder on the floor as much as possible. Your hips should remain in line with your shoulders. Keep the pubic bone moving down. To deepen the twist, move your lower abdomen to the left. Turn your head toward the left and look out over your left hand. Hold for ten to fifteen seconds, breathing evenly. Exhale, bend the knees, and come back to center. Practice on the opposite side.

3. Variation. Practice as in #2, but only bring your knees to the floor; do not straighten your legs.

Benefits: Belly Turning Pose (Jathara Parivartanasana) strengthens and releases the back and opens the hips. It also massages the abdominal organs and firms the abdomen.

BHARADVAJASANA

SIMPLE TWIST

1. Placement. First, sit on your heels as in Diamond Pose (Chapter 8). Then shift your weight to the left, and sit on the floor on your left buttock. Slide your left shin and foot under your right thigh, place your right hand on your left knee. Place your left hand behind you in line with your left thigh.

2. Pose. Inhale and lengthen the spine. Exhale and press down with the hands and turn the torso to the left, rolling the right hip forward. To come more deeply into the twist, inhale and lengthen your spine; exhale and walk your left hand farther back. Maintaining the length of the spine, stretch your right buttock back toward the floor. Hold for ten to fifteen seconds, breathing evenly. Release slowly and practice on the opposite side.

3. Variation. Practice as in #2, but keep your right hip rolled forward and your right buttock off the floor.

4. Aid. Sit as in #1, with the left side of your body six inches away from a wall. Inhale and lengthen your spine; exhale and turn left to face the wall, placing your hands on the wall at shoulder level. As you exhale and turn, push your hands against the wall to assist your coming more deeply into the twist. Repeat on the other side.

Benefits: Simple Twist (Bharadvajasana) increases the flexibility of the entire spine.

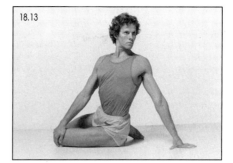

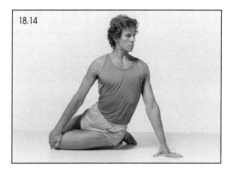

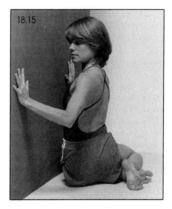

18.13   Simple Twist–with hips down
18.14   Simple Twist–with hip rolled forward
18.15   Simple Twist–at wall

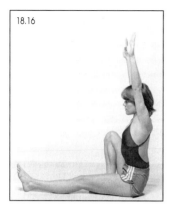

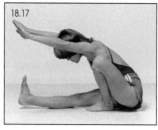

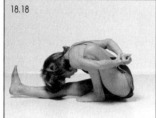

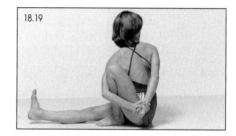

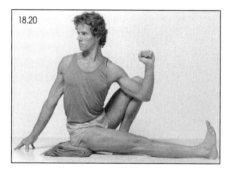

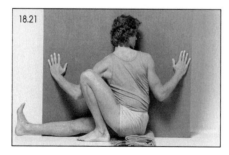

18.16   With arms overhead
18.17   Extending forward
18.18   Seated Twist–hold wrist
18.19   Seated Twist
18.20   Seated Twist–on blanket
18.21   Seated Twist–at wall

MARICHYASANA I

SEATED TWIST

1. Placement. Sit in Staff Pose (Chapter 17). Exhale, bend your left knee, and place your left foot on the floor close to your left sitting bone.

2. Pose. Inhale, lengthen your spine, and raise your arms overhead. Exhale and extend slightly forward as in a forward bend. Wrap your left arm around your left knee and circle your right arm behind you against your back. Clasp your hands. Inhale and lengthen your spine; exhale and turn your torso to the right. As you turn, allow the navel and lower abdominal flesh to come along. Broaden the upper chest. Soften your throat and eyes. Hold for ten to twenty seconds, breathing evenly. Slowly uncoil and then practice on the opposite side.

3. Variation. Sit on one or more firm, folded blankets. Practice as in #2, but do not take hold of your hands. Instead, keep your right fingers on the floor. Bend your left elbow and keep your forearm perpendicular to the floor. Make a fist and, pressing your left elbow against your inner left knee, turn your torso to the right.

4. Aid. Practice as in #2, with the right leg and buttock beside a wall. Bring your left arm in front of your left knee, and place both hands on the wall. Inhale and lengthen your spine; exhale and press your hands against the wall to help you come into the twist. Repeat on the other side.

Caution: This pose is particularly contraindicated for students with herniated discs.

Benefits: Seated Twist (Marichyasana I) tones and massages the abdominal area. It also relieves lower back pain caused by muscular tension.

19
WAKE UP

SUN SALUTATION

The Sun Salutation (Surya Namaskar) is a combination of poses done by moving smoothly from one to the other while coordinating breath with movement (vinyasa). There are many combinations possible; the first version given here is to be practiced in the early stages of learning yoga, the second version is for later on, when you have increased spinal elongation and overall strength.

Before doing Sun Salutation, be sure to practice each of the poses as they were presented earlier. Once you have some understanding of each individual pose in the series, you may wish to use Sun Salutation as a morning warm-up, as its name implies, or as a general warm-up before any athletic activity.

If you look at the poses you can see why Sun Salutation is an excellent warm-up for the total body. The series begins in Mountain Pose, so alignment is established. This is followed by forward bending, groin stretches, and backbending. The arms and wrists are strengthened and stretched in Yoga Push-Up and Upward-Facing Dog Pose. The back is lengthened, the chest opened. By coordinating the inhalation and exhalation with the movement in the poses, awareness is directed to the breath. Practicing the series until it flows

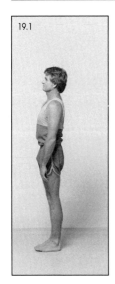

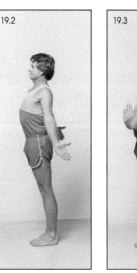

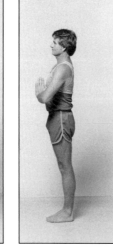

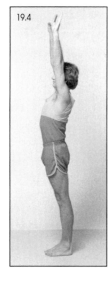

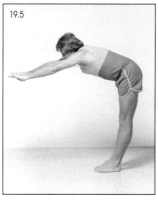

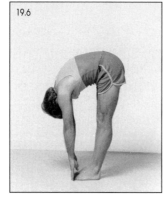

19.1 Mountain Pose
19.2 Mountain Pose–palms out
19.3 Mountain Pose–prayer position
19.4 Mountain Pose–arms overhead
19.5 Standing Forward Bend–coming forward
19.6 Standing Forward Bend

smoothly increases flexibility, strength, and coordination.

Because these versions of Sun Salutation concentrate on one side of the body at a time, you must always balance the body by doing the series twice, first stepping back with one leg, and then for the second time stepping back with your other leg. Also, although the series is meant to be done by moving from one pose to the next with each breath, you can do Sun Salutation more slowly by holding each posture. Use the breath to move into the pose, and then breathe evenly as you hold. It may help you to remember when to inhale and when to exhale if you know, in general, to inhale on backbending movements and exhale on forward bending movements.

SURYA NAMASKAR

SUN SALUTATION I

1. Mountain Pose (Tadasana). Align your body and breathe evenly. Take the time to notice inner sensations.

2. Mountain Pose (Tadasana)–Palms Out. Inhale and turn your palms out. Roll the upper arms out, stretch the fingers down, and lengthen the spine.

3. Prayer Position (Namaste). Exhale and place your palms together in front of your sternum, with your chest broad and your shoulders low.

4. Mountain Pose (Tadasana)–Arms Overhead. Inhale and stretch your arms overhead, with your palms forward. Lengthen from the heels to the fingertips.

5. Standing Forward Bend (Uttanasana). Exhale slowly as you bend forward from your hips, keeping your arms in line with your torso.

6. Complete Forward Bend (Uttanasana). Lifting your buttocks, let your back soften as your hands stretch gently toward the floor.

7. Preparation for Lunge Position. Bend your knees and place your hands on either side of your feet.

8. Lunge Position. Inhale and step your right foot back, turning your toes under as you bend your left leg to form a right angle. Let the right knee come down to the floor as you lengthen the torso out on the left thigh.

9. Plank Position (Chaturanga Dandasana). Check that both hands point directly forward. Breathe evenly. Step your left foot back so you are in a plank position. Stretching out through your heels, activate both thighs. Push the floor away with your hands. Stretch out through the crown of the head and keep the shoulders low, away from the ears.

10. Bent-Knee Push-Up (Chaturanga Dandasana). On an exhalation bend your knees to the floor, and take your feet off the floor. Bending your elbows, lower your torso down with control. Then lie on the floor, straighten your legs, and bring your arms down to your sides.

11. Preparation for Cobra Pose (Bhujangasana). Inhale and lift your head, shoulders, and hands off the floor. Activate your thighs and stretch out through the crown of your head. Do not allow your eyes to roll up toward the ceiling, but keep your gaze soft and look forward.

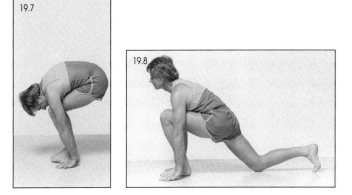

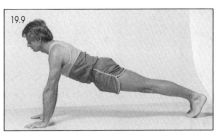

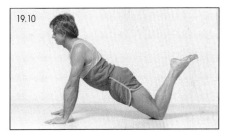

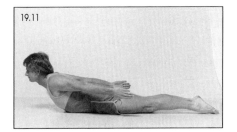

19.7 Lunge Position–preparation
19.8 Lunge Position
19.9 Push-Up Position
19.10 Bent-Knee Push-Up
19.11 Preparation for Cobra Pose

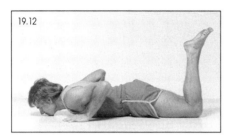

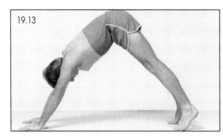

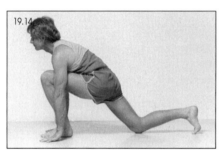

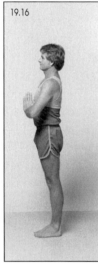

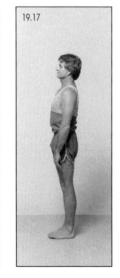

12. Bent-Knee Push-Up (Chaturanga Dandasana). Breathe evenly and place your hands next to your chest. Bend your knees and lift your feet off the floor. Exhale and straighten your arms, lifting your torso off the floor. Inhale and bring your feet back to the floor and curl your toes under.

13. Downward-Facing Dog Pose (Adho Mukha Svanasana). Exhale, straighten your legs, and lift your buttocks so you are in an inverted V. Stay high up on the toes to get more lift in the sitting bones.

14. Lunge Position. Inhale, bend the right leg, and step the right foot forward, placing the foot between the hands. Let your left knee rest on the floor, and lengthen your torso out on your right thigh.

15. Standing Forward Bend (Uttanasana). Exhale, straighten the right leg, and bring the left foot next to the right. Lift your buttocks high, and activate your thighs. Allow your back to lengthen down.

16. Prayer Position (Namaste). Inhale and, with your hands on your hips, lift your torso as a single unit to return to Mountain Pose (Tadasana). Exhale and bring your palms together in front of your sternum. Breathe evenly.

17. Mountain Pose (Tadasana). Lower your arms to your sides. Realign your body and breathe softly and evenly.

Repeat the entire series, moving into and out of the lunges with your left leg first.

19.12 Bent-Knee Push-Up
19.13 Downward-Facing Dog Pose
19.14 Lunge Position
19.15 Standing Forward Bend
19.16 Mountain Pose–prayer position
19.17 Mountain Pose

SURYA NAMASKAR

SUN SALUTATION II

1. Mountain Pose (Tadasana). Align your body and breathe evenly. Take the time to quiet yourself.

2. Mountain Pose (Tadasana)–Palms Out. Inhale and turn your palms out. Lowering your shoulders, stretch your fingers down and lengthen your spine.

3. Prayer Position (Namaste). Exhale and place your palms together in front of your sternum. Broaden the collarbones.

4. Mountain Pose (Tadasana)–Arms Overhead. Inhale and stretch your arms overhead. As your balance and confidence build, look up at your hands. To arch the back, be sure to lengthen the front of the spine and keep the thighs active.

5. Standing Forward Bend (Uttanasana). Exhale slowly as you bend forward from your hips, stretching your arms out from your torso.

6. Standing Forward Bend (Uttanasana). Place your hands on either side of your feet.

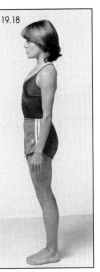

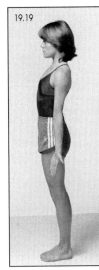

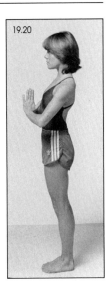

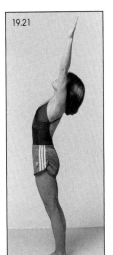

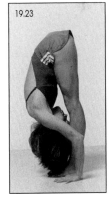

19.18   Mountain Pose
19.19   Mountain Pose–palms out
19.20   Mountain Pose–prayer position
19.21   Mountain Pose–arms overhead
19.22   Standing Forward Bend–bending forward
19.23   Standing Forward Bend–hands beside feet

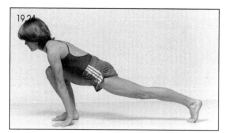

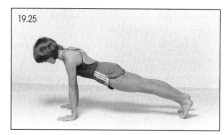

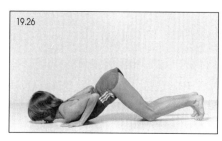

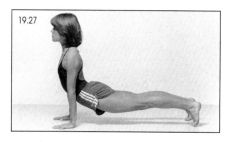

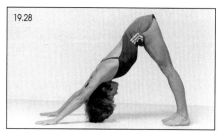

19.24 Lunge Position
19.25 Push-Up Position
19.26 Grasshopper Pose
19.27 Upward-Facing Dog Pose
19.28 Downward-Facing Dog
      Pose

7. Lunge Position. Inhale and step your right foot back, turning your toes under as you bend your left leg to form a right angle. Bring the buttocks down so the body is straight from head to heel. Lengthen your spine and broaden your collarbones.

8. Plank Position (Chaturanga Dandasana). Check that both hands point directly forward. Breathe evenly. Step the left foot back so you are in a plank position. Elongate the elbows, knees, and spine while keeping the throat soft.

9. Grasshopper Pose. Exhale and bend the elbows and knees as you tip the buttocks up. Lower yourself to the floor so your knees, chest, and chin touch the floor simultaneously.

10. Upward-Facing Dog Pose (Urdhva Mukha Svanasana). Inhale, straighten your arms and legs, and come into Upward-Facing Dog Pose. Keep the thighs active and broaden the collarbones to open the chest. Press the floor away from you with your hands. Keep your throat and eyes soft.

11. Downward-Facing Dog Pose (Adho Mukha Svanasana). Exhale, lift your buttocks high, and stretch into Downward-Facing Dog Pose. Stretch your heels down and lengthen your legs.

12. Lunge Position. Inhale, bend the right leg, and step the right foot forward, placing the foot between the hands. Keep your body in a straight line.

13. Standing Forward Bend (Uttanasana). Exhale, straighten the right leg and bring the left foot next to the right. Lift the buttocks high and keep the thighs active.

14. Returning to Mountain Pose (Tadasana). Inhale, place your arms out in front of you, and lift your arms and torso as a single unit to come back up into Mountain Pose, arms up.

15. Prayer Position (Namaste). Exhale and lower your hands into Prayer Position. Breathe evenly.

16. Mountain Pose (Tadasana). Lower your arms to your sides. Realign your body and breathe softly and evenly.

Repeat the entire series, moving into and out of the lunges with your left leg first.

Benefits: Sun Salutation (Surya Namaskar) is an excellent overall warm-up that brings flexibility to the spine and legs, opens the chest, and strengthens the arms and shoulders. It also develops coordination and breath control.

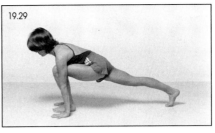

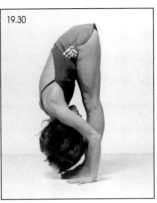

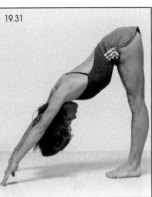

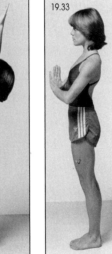

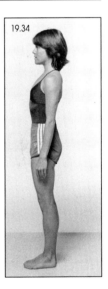

19.29 Lunge Position
19.30 Standing Forward
       Bend–hands beside feet
19.31 Standing Forward
       Bend–arms extended
       forward
19.32 Mountain Pose–arms
       overhead
19.33 Mountain Pose–prayer
       position
19.34 Mountain Pose

20
RELAX AND RENEW

RESTING POSES

For physical, mental, and emotional balance, you need to rest after each and every yoga practice or athletic workout. With the exception of the nerve cells, the entire body is constantly being regenerated: old cells die and new cells replace them. The nerve cells, however, are with you your whole life. Your nervous system, therefore, needs frequent rest. Yoga relaxation allows muscle after muscle to rest, thereby minimizing the bombardment of impulses being conducted by the nervous system. Once you have acquired the knack of it, a ten-minute relaxation can leave you more refreshed than an hour's nap.

Physiologically, resting after a calisthenic workout is essential to eliminate fatigue. As muscles contract, no oxygen is consumed or carbon dioxide produced, so lactic acid content increases. When the muscles are relaxed and oxygen is brought to them via the respiratory system, the lactic acid content decreases. In most physical activities the respiratory system cannot supply adequate oxygen to fully eliminate lactic acid, and so fatigue results. Resting for even a short time will reduce these effects and will probably make an enormous difference in your attitude toward your workout.

Psychologically you need to relax. Tension stores itself in your body. It is seen in a tight belly, clenched jaw, furrowed brow: abundant unnecessary muscle contractions that sap your energy and wear away at your nervous system. But how do you let go, free yourself of what seems to be self-perpetuating tension? Through relaxation! With practice, it can be learned.

First, do some yoga poses to release muscular tension. Then assume a comfortable position (such as the Corpse Pose described in this chapter) in a quiet place. You must then feel inwardly for any areas that are tight. To attain relaxation the mind must first "see" the tension and then allow for its softening.

Relaxation is neither something you can feign nor something you can force; it has to be genuine and pursued patiently or it will elude you. This is why relaxation is the ultimate tool in balancing the body and mind. But the state of relaxation is like quicksilver. With only the slightest wavering, only a moment's wandering of the mind, the muscles can contract and draw you into a tense state again. To relax, both the body and the brain must cooperate. They must be one with the other: yoked. When this happens, you become whole.

Frequent experiences of relaxation will affect other areas of your life, so that as you conduct the business of living, there will be a calmness that underlies all action. Just as tension accumulates in your body, so does calmness. It is manifested in harmony of movement, in an even breath, in a mind capable of concentration and creativity, in a loving spirit. In athletics we call this efficiency, in medicine we call this health, in living we call this comfort, in yoga we call this balance.

So relaxation has lots to offer if only you will take the time to do it. Ten to twenty minutes is most often suggested. How about doing one to two minutes at first? When doing Corpse Pose, begin by just focusing on your breath. Watch it, don't change it. Feel your body grow heavier. Gravity is real; it draws every cell in your body toward the center of the Earth. Feel yourself loosen as you let go. Then begin at your toes and work methodically up your body, feeling the toes, the soles of the feet, each leg, the torso, and so on, up to the crown of the head. There's nothing magical about relaxation. With time and proper attention, it's yours.

VAJRASANA, VARIATION

CHILD'S POSE

1. Placement. Sit on your blanket or mat in Diamond Pose (Chapter 8), with your knees together, and your feet parallel and slightly apart. Inhale and lengthen your spine.

2. Pose. Bend at your hips and stretch your torso forward until your forehead rests on the floor. Tuck the chin slightly to lengthen the neck. Place your hands alongside your torso, palms up. Relax your face, neck, shoulders, arms, hands, and abdomen. Feel gravity draw you toward the earth. Breathe quietly.

3. Aid. If sitting in this position is difficult and you are unable to relax, place a cushion between your feet and buttocks. Do not use a cushion so large that the body weight goes too far forward onto the forehead. Let the weight be distributed evenly from your head to your toes. If your head does not touch the floor, place another cushion under your head.

4. Aid. If you are tight in the groins, place a rolled towel across both groins. Pull back on the towel as you bend the torso over it. Most pain is caused by compression, and this aid may help to make space and relieve the pressure.

Benefits: Child's Pose (Vajrasana) releases tension in the lower back. It is also particularly useful after sitting forward bends and backbends.

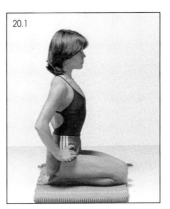

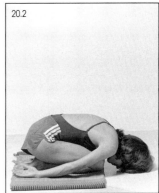

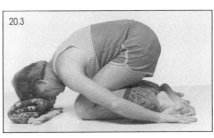

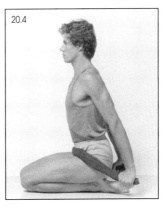

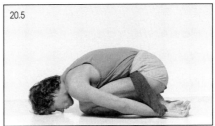

20.1   Child's Pose–placement
20.2   Child's Pose
20.3   Child's Pose–with support
20.4   Child's Pose with towel
       across groin–placement
20.5   Child's Pose with towel
       across groin

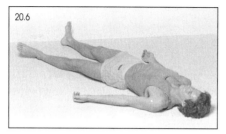

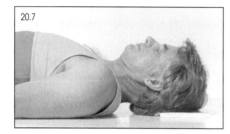

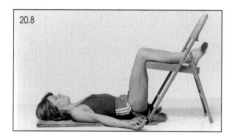

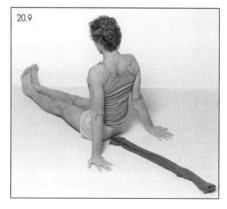

20.6   Corpse Pose
20.7   Corpse Pose–lift under head
20.8   Corpse Pose–legs resting on
        chair
20.9   Corpse Pose–towel under
        spine

SAVASANA

CORPSE POSE

1. Placement. Lie on your back in Mountain Pose. Separate your feet about eighteen inches apart, and allow them to fall out to the sides. Place your hands about a foot away from your torso, palms turned up. Allow the eyes to close.

2. Pose. Lie still. Breathe, releasing any tension with each exhalation. Let your body sink back toward the floor. Keeping your eyes closed, direct your eyeballs toward your heart. Keep the jaw relaxed so the teeth are not touching, and the tongue is broad in the mouth. As your body softens, it will lengthen. Note how your mind wanders, and gently bring your attention back to your body and breath. Hold for five to twenty minutes.

3. Aid. If your chin is higher than your forehead in this pose, place a slim book, folded towel, or cushion under the back of your head. Raise your head until your chin is parallel to the floor.

4. Aid. If your back aches for any reason, place your lower legs on a chair, or simply bend your knees and place both feet on the floor. Lifting or bending the legs in this way usually will relieve any discomfort. If discomfort persists do a gentle Crocodile Twist (Chapter 18), followed by Knees-to-Chest Pose (Chapter 12), and then again Corpse Pose. Let go, rest.

5. Aid. To gently stretch the chest, place a vertically folded towel or blanket so you are supported from the waist to the head. You may also need to place another folded towel under your head.

6. Aid. If bright lights are unavoidable, put a folded towel across your eyes so your eyes can fully relax.

Benefits: Corpse Pose (Savasana) relaxes and refreshes all systems of the body. It also brings the body, mind, and spirit into balance.

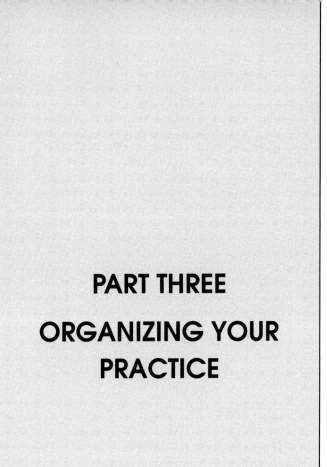

PART THREE

ORGANIZING YOUR PRACTICE

21
BASIC PRACTICE GUIDE

The core poses in this book include the standing poses, Standing Forward Bend, Downward-Facing Dog Pose, Upward-Facing Dog Pose, Hero Pose, Shoulderstand, Plough Pose, and Corpse Pose. Practicing these poses strengthens and stretches the legs, opens the hips, lengthens the spine, and rejuvenates the body. Although the other poses and stretches presented here have intrinsic value and many help to prepare you for the core poses, it is these core poses that should be the focus of an ongoing, health-giving practice, particularly for the first couple of years. So effective practice consists of an exploration of your body mostly in these core poses. It's as simple as that. (See Chapter 22 for a specific practice schedule.)

Unfortunately, what I often see is that people take a few stretches from this book, such as Achilles Tendon and Calf Stretch or Runner's Warm-Up, and use them simply to prevent injury. This method may be effective in preventing a specific injury, but it deprives you of an overall increase in well-being. Gravity, stress, and improper exercise gradually produce compression. I want you to know that if you follow a yoga program, you will probably feel much better, better in a way that it's hard to describe, because of the skeletal extension and muscular flexibility you will gain. Actually, I can think of a way to describe how you probably will feel: younger.

It is essential to practice the standing poses. From what I've observed of athletes, they often take the time to stretch their legs, but do not remember to lengthen their spines. Many stretches for the feet and legs are an inherent part of the standing poses, and because the spine can lengthen in these poses they are incredibly efficient. Once you take some time to understand them, they are yours forever.

Spend your first practice session exploring the information presented in Chapters 4, 5, and 6. Read these chapters as many times as is necessary to incorporate the information into your practice routine. Once you understand this material, you are ready to organize your practice. Several possible strategies follow. They are based on a six-day practice sequence (rest on the seventh) of thirty to forty minutes. I am assuming that you, the reader, are probably busy with work at home and in the outside world, and are interested in yoga as a way to feel good (even great) and as a holistic way to support yourself in any sport you do for health and fun. (If you become interested in developing a more intense practice, you can consult B. K. S. Iyengar's *Light on Yoga.* See Chapter 25, "Resources.")

Initial Strategy

The best strategy initially is to concentrate on practicing the first seven standing poses: Mountain Pose, Tree Pose, Triangle Pose, Warrior Pose II, Side Angle Pose, Intense Side Stretch Pose, and Warrior Pose I. Understanding these poses is so important that it is wise in the beginning to take almost an entire practice session to work on a single standing pose. For example, you may want to first do the complete pose, and then experiment with each variation and aid for that specific pose. Experimenting may reveal, for example, that your legs are tight, so you would turn to hamstring stretches and work there. Working in this way will enable you to follow your own needs and allow your body to become your guide.

In any given week do not introduce any more than three new standing poses into your practice. Standing poses are complex; they affect the whole body. So take the time to understand, to explore, and to allow your body to absorb what you have learned.

Here is a sample outline for the first week of practice:

Day One
Preliminaries
      Squaring the feet
      Lifting the kneecaps
      Activating the thighs
      Pelvic tilting
      Elongating the spine
      Aligning the shoulders
      Placement of the head
Mountain Pose
Jumping
Corpse Pose

Day Two
Lifting the kneecaps
Mountain Pose
      Lying on back (#6, aid)
Tree Pose
      Complete Tree Pose
      Arms stretched overhead (#3, variation)
      Back against wall (#4, aid)
You may discover that your hips are tight; if so, turn to Chapter 9 and do Bound Angle Pose. Because you know you're tight, you can begin with one of the aids, for example, #4: sitting on one or more folded blankets with your back against a wall.
Corpse Pose

Day Three
Lifting the kneecaps
Mountain Pose
Tree Pose
      Arms stretched overhead (#3, variation)
      Back against wall (#4, aid)
You may discover that your shoulders are tight; if so, turn to Chapter 14 and practice Chest Opener.
Triangle Pose (just experiment with complete pose)
Bound Angle Pose
Corpse Pose

Day Four
Activating the thighs
Mountain Pose
      Lying on back (#6, aid)
Chest Opener
Mountain Pose
Jumping

Triangle Pose

 Hand on groin (#3, variation)

 Heel against wall (#4, aid)

 Complete pose

You may discover that the backs of your legs are stiff, so turn to Chapter 10 and do Beginner's Hamstring Stretch.

Corpse Pose

Day Five

Pelvic tilting (note where the spine is longest)

Lifting the kneecaps (note where the legs are strongest)

Mountain Pose (strong legs with a long spine)

Chest Opener

Tree Pose

Mountain Pose

Jumping

Triangle Pose

Beginner's Hamstring Stretch

Corpse Pose

Day Six

Review preliminaries

Mountain Pose

Tree Pose

 Back against wall (#4, aid)

Chest Opener

Triangle Pose

 Complete Triangle Pose

 Back against wall (#5, aid)

Beginner's Hamstring Stretch

Bound Angle Pose

 Back against wall (#4, aid)

Staff Pose

 Legs up the wall (#4, aid)

Corpse Pose

Day Seven

Rest

Working carefully, as described in the sample outline of the first week, it is likely that you will take at least eight to ten weeks just to introduce yourself to the first seven standing poses, all the time adding stretches and poses as your need or interest arises. In the list that follows is information about the different types of stretches you may need to understand and execute each standing pose.

Mountain Pose requires spinal elongation.

Tree Pose requires hip and shoulder stretches.

Triangle Pose requires leg stretches, flexible hips, and slight twists.

Warrior Pose II requires hip stretches and thigh strength.

Side Angle Pose requires all that is named in the preceding poses.

Intense Side Stretch Pose requires an understanding of forward bending, as well as hand, wrist, and shoulder stretches.

Warrior Pose I requires foot and lower leg stretches, and a preliminary understanding of backbending.

When you begin to feel familiar with the standing poses, start adding to your practice Downward-Facing Dog Pose (Chapter 12), and Locust Pose and Preparation for Cobra Pose (Chapter 15). Proceed to a careful exploration of Shoulderstand and Plough Pose by reading Chapter 16 again. Begin practice of Shoulderstand at the wall, so you are well supported. Be sure to start each practice with two or three standing poses to warm up, and particularly to elongate the spine, before attempting Shoulderstand. Also begin to incorporate stretches preparing the legs for Hero Pose if you haven't already done so (Chapter 8).

This first strategy, then, is to understand the essential poses for basic overall flexibility and spinal extension. I emphasize the understanding of the poses, because it may take decades to master the poses. You see, it's not important to do these poses as they are pictured in the complete pose. It is imperative that you practice at the level of your ability: that's the complete pose for you. Any straining or pushing is not yoga, and is detrimental to your health and well-being.

Once you have experimented with this initial strategy, there are other ways of proceeding.

From-the-Ground-Up Strategy

This strategy is to practice from the ground up. Start with stretches for the feet and legs, and work right up the body. This parallels roughly the way this book is laid out. Until you become familiar with the poses and your individual needs you can proceed by doing the first pose in each chapter one day, the second pose in each chapter the next day, and so on. It may take two days or more to actually complete the poses from feet to head, so for the first couple of years, if you need to break up the series, be sure to warm up each day with at least two standing poses. Working this way is progressive; the poses, in general, get harder, and you won't avoid any challenging areas or favor certain poses.

Rotation Strategy

Another strategy popularly used is to practice certain types of poses on specific days. Following are suggestions on how to proceed. Again, for the first couple of years, be sure to begin all practice sessions with at least two standing poses. Usually this fits in easily with the theme for the day. For example, on the day you do twists, you might begin naturally with Triangle Pose and Revolved Triangle Pose. On the day you are do backbends, it would be appropriate to start with Warrior Pose I and Warrior Pose III. Be sure to end each practice with a resting pose.

Elementary Rotation Practice

Monday	Standing poses (Chapter 7)
Tuesday	Feet, leg, hamstring, and hip stretches (Chapters 8, 9, 10)
Wednesday	Abdominal strengtheners, standing forward bends, and twists (Chapters 11, 13, 18)
Thursday	Shoulder and arm stretches, inverted poses (Chapters 14, 16)
Friday	Back stretches and backbends (Chapters 12, 15)
Saturday	Hip, hamstring, and back stretches, Sun Salutation I (Chapters 9, 10, 12, 19)
Sunday	Rest

Advanced Rotation Practice

Monday	Standing poses (Chapter 7)
Tuesday	Forward-bending poses, standing and seated (Chapters 13, 17)
Wednesday	Feet, leg, and hip stretches, abdominal strengtheners, twisting poses (Chapters 8, 9, 11, 18)
Thursday	Hamstring, shoulder and arm stretches, inverted poses (Chapters 10, 14, 16)
Friday	Back stretches and backbends (Chapters 12, 15)
Saturday	Hip, hamstring, and back stretches, Sun Salutation II (Chapters 9, 10, 12, 19)
Sunday	Rest

Responsive Strategy

As you become more familiar with the poses and with your own body, yoga will become a way for you to respond to yourself. You will begin to notice how you feel, and do poses that are appropriate to your physical or emotional state.

In the first instance, you might notice that you have some persistent tightnesses or weaknesses. The poses you practice in the Initial Strategy section will probably make you aware of them. So you may want to focus your practice on these areas for a while, making sure you approach these areas with curiosity and compassion. The reason they are out of balance in the first place is because these areas already have been stressed; being aggressive will not help. But they do, in fact, need your attention, which is why your body is giving you signals. It's important to respond.

Another way tightness and weakness can be perceived is to notice where your skeletal system collapses. One way you can tell is by noticing wrinkles. For example, if you have folds or wrinkles on the front of the torso, you are tight in the front and weak in the back. To counteract this tendency, build in spinal elongation by practicing back strengtheners and backbends, in combination with the standing poses. Conversely, if you have folds in the back (ask a partner to look there, use a mirror to see there, or explore there by feeling with your hands), you are tight in the back and weak in the front. To counteract this tendency, strengthen the abdomen and stretch the back, again in combination with the standing poses.

Another responsive approach to practice focuses on how you are feeling. Shoulderstand, forward bending poses, and twists have a calming effect on the body. Say you did something athletic in the evening and as a result feel too keyed up to go to sleep, but you have a commitment the next day for which you'd like to be fresh. No problem. Spend twenty minutes in calming poses, focusing on what you are feeling, and you're likely to fall asleep soon after. Or during the day, say you run at noon and have a presentation in the afternoon, and you don't want to be overstimulated. Take some time for forward bends and a twist or two, and you probably will have the desired result.

Conversely, standing poses and backbending poses tend to energize. If your energy is low and you need to be more energtic, do some backbends and usually you'll feel much peppier. The poses you do don't have to be intense. A few minutes in Chest Opener and Camel Pose (#3, aid) are good starters, and could be done easily in office clothes. Of course, if you have the time and the appropriate environment, standing poses in combination with backbends would probably give you a more sustained effect.

In time you will not have to decide logically where you need to stretch; you will be able to feel what needs attention. If you have been busy, distracted, or stressed, you may have to begin with a few stretches to reintroduce yourself to yourself, but then just follow what each pose reveals. This is how you take care of yourself: you give yourself what you need. Remember, teachers and books will come and go, but you will always be with yourself.

22
CORE PROGRAM

Here are basic poses to keep a minimal amount of stretch in the major muscles and openness in the joints of the body. Because each of these poses has aids and variations, you can use this program no matter how flexible you may be. Be sure to add to this list those poses you have found that are essential to keep your tight spots pliable. This list is purposely short so that it is practical for you to do regularly.

Mountain Pose
Triangle Pose
Side Angle Pose
Standing Forward Bend
Downward-Facing Dog Pose
Upward-Facing Dog Pose
Squat Series I–IV
Hero Pose
Leg Lifts
Shoulderstand
Plough Pose
Knees-to-Chest Pose
Progressive Hamstring Stretch or Supine Hand-to-
    Foot Pose
Bound Angle Pose
Seated Forward Bend
Crocodile Twist
Corpse Pose

23
SUGGESTED ROUTINE FOR BEFORE AND AFTER RUNNING

Practice this routine using aids and variations as needed. After long-distance running, wait at least two hours before inverting the body in any way.

Mountain Pose
Triangle Pose
Side Angle Pose
Downward-Facing Dog Pose
Squat Series I–IV
Hero Pose
Runner's Warm-Up
Walk/Run/Walk
Doorknob Stretch I, with or without a partner
Doorknob Stretch II
Standing Groin Stretch
Hero Pose
Wall Hang
Spread-Foot Forward Bend
Downward-Facing Dog Pose
Bound Angle Pose, at the wall (#4, aid)
Open Angle Pose, at the wall (#5, aid)
Shoulderstand, with or without the wall (#4, aid)
Plough Pose, with or without the wall (#3, aid)
Crocodile Twist
Corpse Pose

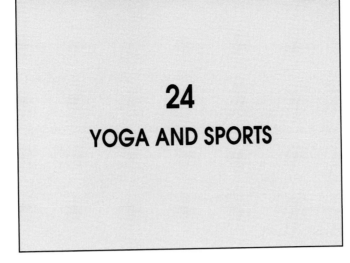

24
YOGA AND SPORTS

Everyone involved in sports can benefit enormously by regular (at least four times a week) practice of the standing poses, so they are recommended across the board. The standing poses lengthen the spine and balance the feet, legs, and hips through the combination of strengthening and lengthening. The poses and stretches that follow are additional suggestions to counteract imbalances inherent in some sports, for example, one-sided sports such as tennis.

Backpacking
Standing poses.

For flexibility: Progressive Hamstring Stretch, all forward bends, back stretches, all feet and ankle poses, all shoulder and arm poses, and backbends.

For strength: Chair Pose, Downward-Facing Dog Pose, Upward-Facing Dog Pose, and Sun Salutation I or Sun Salutation II.

Ballet and Modern Dancing
Standing poses.

For flexibility: Pelvic tilting, with attention to the position where the spine is longest is important. (In recent ballet history there has been an emphasis on tucking the pelvis down, resulting in an overly flat spine.) Practice all standing poses with attention to alignment of the feet. Although ballet is danced with the feet turned out, dancers need to recognize this as a basic misalignment and practice intelligently so the feet are not turned out in their daily activities. Doorknob Stretch for Achilles and Calves, Achilles Tendon and Calf Stretch, Squat Series, Hero Pose, and back stretches.

For strength: Upward-Facing Dog Pose, Downward-Facing Dog Pose, and inverted poses.

Basketball

Do the poses recommended in Chapter 23, "Suggested Routine for Before and After Running." In addition, place a strong emphasis on standing poses, with careful attention to the knees. Do lots of back stretches, and focus on carefully developing a practice to include long Shoulderstands. Continually work to keep the shoulder joints flexible. If the shoulders get tight, the back compensates by overarching, and this puts strain on the lower back. Build time in Chair Pose.

Bicycling

Standing poses.

For flexibility: Practice the forward bends, focusing on bending at the hip joints, and remember to sit this way on your bike. Most bikers hunch over to reach the handlebars. When sitting on your bike, tilt the pelvis forward by sitting on the front edge of the sitting bones, and elongate the front of your torso so the spine is lengthened. If this is impossible or uncomfortable, have your bike adjusted by a professional, who will fit it to your proportions. Practice Chest Opener, Hero Pose and its variations, all groin stretches, back stretches, backbends, and Shoulderstand.

For strength: Chair Pose, Yoga Push-Ups, Preparation for Cobra Pose, Locust Pose, and Shoulderstand.

Boating

Standing poses.

For flexibility: Handclasp Shoulder Stretch, Wrist Stretch, back stretches, all forward bends, all backbends, twists, and groin stretches. Because boating requires a lot of bending over, be sure to practice forward bending, so that you will learn to habitually bend forward from the hips. This will relieve and prevent back discomfort and injuries.

For strength: Preparation for Cobra Pose, Locust Pose, and Shoulderstand.

Bowling

Standing poses.

For flexibility: Chest Opener, back stretches, shoulder and arm stretches, and twists.

For strength: Downward-Facing Dog Pose, Upward-Facing Dog Pose, and Yoga Push-Ups.

Cross-Country Skiing

Standing poses.

For flexibility: Hero Pose and its variations, groin stretches, forward bends, backbends, all hamstring stretches, Squat Series, back stretches, Chest Opener, and Cow's Face Pose.

For strength: Preparation for Cobra Pose, Locust Pose, inverted poses, and Sun Salutation I or II.

Downhill Skiing

Standing poses.

For flexibility: Groin stetches, hip and inner leg stretches, back stretches, twists, and Chest Opener.

For strength: Chair Pose, arm strengtheners, Preparation for Cobra Pose, Locust Pose, and inverted poses.

Folk and Square Dancing

Standing poses.

For flexibility: Progressive Hamstring Stretch, all poses for feet, knees, and lower legs, and back stretches. Practice all variations of Downward-Facing Dog Pose. All the twisting poses, particularly Revolved Triangle Pose, with careful attention to alignment. Wrist Stretch and Cow's Face Pose.

For strength: Downward-Facing Dog Pose, Upward-Facing Dog Pose, Yoga Push-Ups, Shoulderstand.

Golf

Because they twist while swinging, lower back pain is a common complaint of golfers. To remedy this, pay careful attention to alignment in all poses and learn to twist correctly. Read the introduction to Chapter 18, "Revolve and Resolve: Twisting Poses," carefully. As you position yourself before you swing, be sure you are bending forward at the hips, not at the waist. Chapter 13, "Suspension: Standing Forward Bends," will give you good practice at this important movement.

Standing poses.

For flexibility: Handclasp Shoulder Stretch, Wrist

Stretch, back stretches, all hamstring stretches, all forward bending poses, and all twisting poses.

For strength: Chair Pose, Preparation for Cobra Pose, Locust Pose, Downward-Facing Dog Pose, and Upward-Facing Dog Pose.

Gymnastics

Standing poses.

For flexibility: All of the poses in the core program (Chapter 22) will increase your flexibility. The important ingredient for the successful practice of yoga is your mental attitude. There is no spirit of competition here. Flexibility will come with patient, persistent practice. Pay attention to physical sensations and not to results.

For strength: It is important to practice the standing poses with attention to alignment and spinal elongation. The standing poses in particular balance the body between strength and flexibility, which is especially important for female gymnasts, who tend to be more flexible than male gymnasts, and who sometimes get overly stretched. If you are overly stretched you are more flexible than strong, which is as dangerous as being too tight; it's just not as common. Take special care in backbending. Gymnasts often overwork the lumbar area by bending exclusively in the lower back. Be sure to elongate the lumbar as you backbend, and extend the arching into the upper back. Stretch the spine, don't just fold over it.

Horseback Riding

Standing Poses.

For flexibility: Back stretches, Progressive Hamstring Stretch, Bound Angle Pose, Open Angle Pose, all groin stretches, foot stretches, particularly Achilles Tendon and Calf Stretch and Hero Pose and its variations, and twists.

For strength: Yoga Push-Ups, stomach strengtheners, Locust Pose, Preparation for Cobra Pose, Downward-Facing Dog Pose, Upward-Facing Dog Pose, and Shoulderstand.

Ice Skating

Standing poses.

For flexibility: Back stretches and all poses for feet, knees, and lower legs.

For strength: Downward-Facing Dog Pose, Upward-

Facing Dog Pose, Sun Salutation I or Sun Salutation II, Shoulderstand, and Plough Pose.

Racquet Sports

It is difficult to balance when playing racquet sports, because they are so one sided. For true balance, it would be necessary to play equal amounts of time using the dominant arm and the nondominant arm. So stretch your dominant side more, and strengthen the nondominant side as much as possible.

Standing poses.

For flexibility: All forward bends, particularly Spread-Foot Forward Bend, with the arms overhead (#4, variation), all shoulder and arm stretches, Wrist Stretch, Squat Series (all four poses), Hero Pose and all its variations, stretches for lower legs, hips, and thighs, back stretches, and backbends. To help prevent tennis elbow, do Plough Pose with the fingers interlaced (#4, variation) or while holding a pole or towel (#5, aid), frequently.

For strength: Chair Pose, Upward-Facing Dog Pose, Downward-Facing Dog Pose.

Running

See Chapter 23, "Suggested Routine for Before and After Running."

Soccer

Standing poses.

For flexibility: Do the poses in Chapter 23, "Suggested Routine for Befre and After Running," particularly Hero Pose and its variations, groin stretches, Downward-Facing Dog Pose, and all back stretches. Do Shoulderstand and Plough Pose to stretch the neck after heading.

For strength: Chair Pose, Downward-Facing Dog Pose, Upward-Facing Dog Pose, and Sun Salutation I or Sun Salutation II.

Softball

Standing poses.

For flexibility: Hip stretches, shoulder stretches, and all the stretches for the spine. Work to understand lengthening the spine while twisting.

For strength: Chair Pose, Downward-Facing Dog Pose, Upward-Facing Dog Pose, and Sun Salutation I or Sun Salutation II.

Swimming

Standing poses.

For flexibility: Achilles Tendon and Calf Stretch, Squat Series I–IV, Hero Pose and all its variations (especially good for ankles and feet), twists, and stretches for shoulders and arms. Flexible shoulders can really give a swimmer the competitive edge. Flexibility here means you can reach farther and this affects everything, from the way you enter the water to your touch at the end of the pool.

For strength: Inverted poses, Downward-Facing Dog Pose, and Upward-Facing Dog Pose.

Volleyball

Standing poses.

For flexibility: Shoulder stretches, Chest Opener, Wrist Stretch, and inverted poses.

For strength: Chair Pose and Sun Salutation I or II.

Walking

Standing poses.

For flexibility: Forward bends, stretches for the feet, and all spine lengtheners.

For strength: Downward-Facing Dog Pose, Upward-Facing Dog Pose, Yoga Push-Ups, Leg Lifts, Yoga Sit-Ups.

Water Skiing

Standing poses.

For flexibility: Stretches for shoulders and arms, poses for feet, knees, and lower legs, back stretches, backbends, and twists.

For strength: Upward-Facing Dog Pose, Downward-Facing Dog Pose, and Shoulderstand.

Weight Lifting

Standing poses.

For flexibility: Do all back stretches regularly. Work carefully to understand spinal elongation in twisting positions. Twisting compresses the spine, so if you are out of alignment and twisting with weights, you are putting yourself in a precarious situation. Also, be sure to do stretches for the hamstrings and shoulders, because if you lose flexibility here, the spine must compensate.

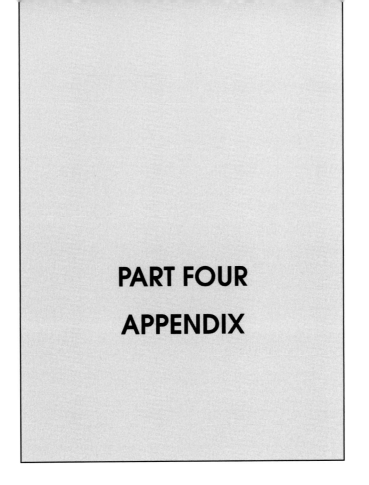

PART FOUR

APPENDIX

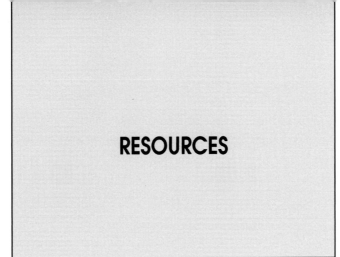

RESOURCES

B O O K S

Light on Yoga
B.K.S. Iyengar (New York: Schocken, 1979)
A comprehensive guidebook to Hatha Yoga, including 602 photographs and detailed explanations on how to practice.

Light on Pranayama
B.K.S. Iyengar (New York: Crossroad, 1981)
A clear, detailed account of the yogic art of breathing, together with a comprehensive background of yoga philosophy.

Light on the Yoga Sutras of Patanjali
B.K.S. Iyengar
(San Francisco: Aquarian/HarperCollins, 1993)
A fresh translation of Patanjali's philosophy and the art of practicing yoga.

Tree of Yoga
B.K.S. Iyengar
(Boston: Shambhala, 1989)
A master of Hatha Yoga offers thoughts on many subjects: health and the healing arts, asana practice and teaching, Patanjali's *Yoga Sutras,* and more.

Yoga: A Gem for Women
Geeta S. Iyengar
(Spokane, Wash.: Timeless Books, 1983)
A comprehensive approach to Hatha Yoga, including special instructions for menstruation and pregnancy.

Back Care Basics
Mary Pullig Schatz, M.D.
(Berkeley, Calif.: Rodmell Press, 1992)
Learn practical ways to heal your back, restructure your body, and manage stress with a doctor's gentle yoga program for back and neck pain relief.

Relax and Renew
Judith Lasater, Ph.D., P.T.
(Berkeley, Calif.: Rodmell Press, 1995)
Practice restorative yoga: the supported poses and breathing techniques that help ease the effects of stress. Includes programs for back pain, headaches, insomnia; a special section for women; and more.

How to Use Yoga
Mira Mehta
(Berkeley, Calif.: Rodmell Press, 1998)
Explore basic poses, their variations, and learn how to sequence your yoga practice with this unique beginner's guide in the style of B.K.S. Iyengar.

Yoga for Pregnancy
Sandra Jordan
(New York: St. Martin's Press, 1989)
A guidebook of 92 poses to help pregnant women adjust to the demands of labor, birth, and motherhood.

MAGAZINES

The Journal of the International Association of Yoga Therapists
20 Sunnyside Ave., Suite A243
Mill Valley, CA 94941–1928
To subscribe, call 415/332–2478
http://www.yoganet.com
Articles, essays, interviews, and book and video reviews from experts in yoga therapeutics.

Yoga International
RR 1, Box 407
Honesdale, PA 18431–9718
To subscribe, call 800/253–6243
YImag@epix.net
Articles and interviews on yoga philosophy, poses, breathing techniques, meditation, personal growth, and more. Annual feature: *Guide to Yoga Teachers and Classes,* a special supplement to the December/January issue.

Yoga Journal
2054 University Ave., Suite 600
Berkeley, CA 94704–1082
To subscribe, call 800/436–9642
http://www.yogajournal.com
Body/mind approaches to personal and spiritual development, such as Hatha Yoga, meditation, holistic health, and more. Annual feature: *Yoga Teachers Directory,* in the July/August issue; also available as a booklet.

VIDEOS

Yoga Journal's Yoga Practice Series
Patricia Walden and Rodney Yee
(Santa Monica, Calif.: Living Arts)
For beginning and developing students, this award-winning series is uniquely designed to allow you to create your own pesonal practice session: for Beginners, for Flexibility, for Strength, for Relaxation, for Energy, for Meditation, and Remedies for Natural Healing. Seven tapes; 60–80 minutes each; VHS/BETA/PAL. To order, call 800/254-8464; http://www.livingarts.com.

AUDIO

Relaxation
Mary Pullig Schatz, M.D.
(Nashville, Tenn.: Physical Medicine Associates)
Visualization techniques especially suitable for those with asthma, hypertension, or other conditions affecting the circulatory and respiratory systems. 60 minutes. Distributed by Rodmell Press, $9.95, plus $5.00 s/h. Calif. residents add sales tax. To order, call 800/841–3123; RodmellPrs@aol.com.

PROPS

United States

Hugger-Mugger Yoga Products
31 W. Gregson Ave.
Salt Lake City, UT 84115–3726
800/473–4888
http://www.yogacentral.com/hugger

Living Arts
2434 Main St.
Santa Monica, CA 90405–3516
800/254–8464
http://www.livingarts.com

Rodmell Press Yoga Practice Essentials
2147 Blake St.
Berkeley, CA 94704–2715
800/841–3123
RodmellPrs@aol.com

Canada

Half Moon Yoga Props
2–2137 W. First Ave.
Vancouver, B.C. V6K 1E7
604/731–7099

HOW TO FIND A YOGA TEACHER

Contact these Iyengar yoga associations for more information about yoga, a teacher in your area, and teacher training programs.

United States

**B.K.S. Iyengar Yoga National Association
of the United States, Inc.**
P.O. Box 79561
Atlanta, GA 30357–7561
800/889–9642
http://www.iyoga.com/IYNAUS/

Canada

Canadian Iyengar Yoga Teachers Association
c/o 2428 Yonge St.
Toronto, Ont. M4P 2H4
416/482–1333

ABOUT THE AUTHOR

Jean Couch lives in the San Francisco Bay Area, and teaches yoga at The Balance Center in Palo Alto, California, as well as workshops and retreats throughout the United States. She has written numberous articles on Hatha Yoga and athletics in *Runner's World, Yoga Journal,* and other periodicals.

Correspondence to the author can be addressed to: Jean Couch, Rodmell Press, 2147 Blake St., Berkeley, CA 94704–2715.

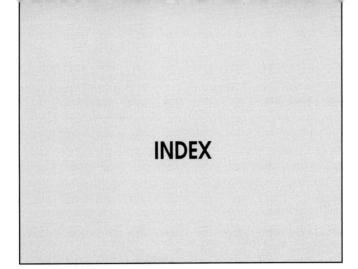

INDEX

POSES
BY CHAPTER

POSES
IN ALPHABETICAL ORDER

DEAR READER,

Our intention is to publish yoga books and tapes that you can *really* use in your practice. To help us learn more about you, your yoga practice, and what you would like us to publish in the future, please complete this questionnaire. We will send you a copy of our latest catalog. Your input is valued and much appreciated.

—Rodmell Press

Name_____

Address _____

City_____State_____Zip_____

Age ❏ 18–24 ❏ 25–49 ❏ 50+
     ❏ Female ❏ Male

Occupation _____

If you're a yoga teacher:

What style of yoga do you teach? _____

How many classes do you teach per week? _____

Do you work with a special population? _____

Would you like to receive information
about selling Rodmell Press books
to your students? ❏ Yes ❏ No

Do you plan to teach yoga? ❏ Yes ❏ No

What brought you to yoga? _____
_____
_____

How did you hear about *The Runner's Yoga Book?* _____
_____
_____

Where did you purchase it? _____
_____

When? _____ Price? _____

Was it a gift? _____

What do you think of it? _____

_____

_____

_____

Please check the following areas of yoga that interest you:

❏ anatomy/kinesiology

❏ back care

❏ breathing/pranayama

❏ children

❏ designing a daily practice

❏ diet/recipes

❏ immune system

❏ meditation

❏ menstruation/menopause

❏ philosophy (*Sutras,* etc.)

❏ pregnancy/childbirth/postpartum

❏ relaxation techniques

❏ restorative poses

❏ sports

❏ stress

❏ teacher training

❏ use of props

❏ women's needs

❏ other (please specify) _____

Send to
Rodmell Press
2147 Blake St.
Berkeley, CA 94704–2715

FROM THE PUBLISHER

Rodmell Press publishes books and tapes on the practice of yoga. In the *Bhagavadgita* it is written, "Yoga is skill in action." It is our hope that our books will help our readers develop a more skillful yoga practice—one that brings peace to their daily lives and to the Earth.

We thank our friends and colleagues whose support, encouragement, and practical advice have sustained us in our efforts. In particular, we are grateful to Reb Anderson, B.K.S. Iyengar, and Yvonne Rand for their inspiration.

Our titles are distributed to bookstores and libraries by S.C.B. Distributors, 15608 S. New Century Dr., Gardena, CA 90248; 800/729–6423; 310/532–9400; 310/532–7001 (fax).

If you are a yoga teacher and would like to make our books and tapes available to your students, write or call us for information on quantity discounts.

For a free copy of our catalog and to receive information on future titles, please send us your name and address.

Rodmell Press
2147 Blake St.
Berkeley, CA 94704–2715

800/841–3123 (order)
510/841–3123 (vox)
510/841–3191 (fax)
RodmellPrs@aol.com

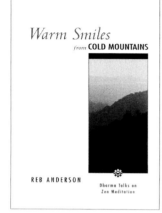
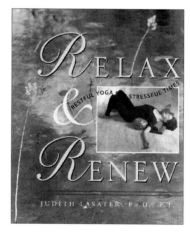
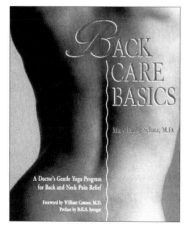